DASH DIET COOKBOOK FOR BEGINNERS 2024

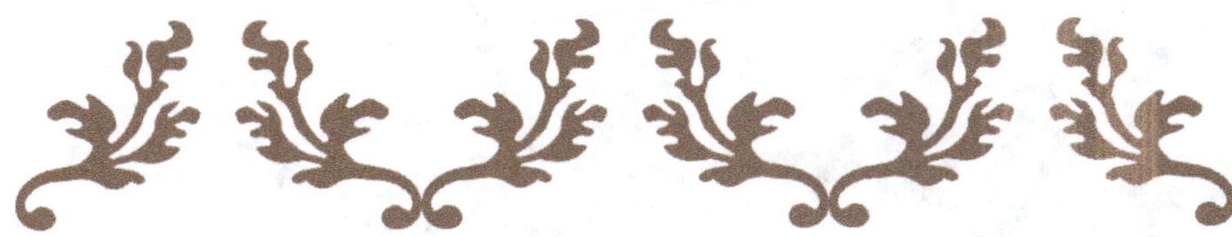

Unlock Easy Tasty Recipes, Discover the Secrets to Lower Blood Pressure and Improve Well-Being, Cut Down on Kitchen Time, Including Full Color Images, health, And Meal Plan

JAMES MCALLISTER

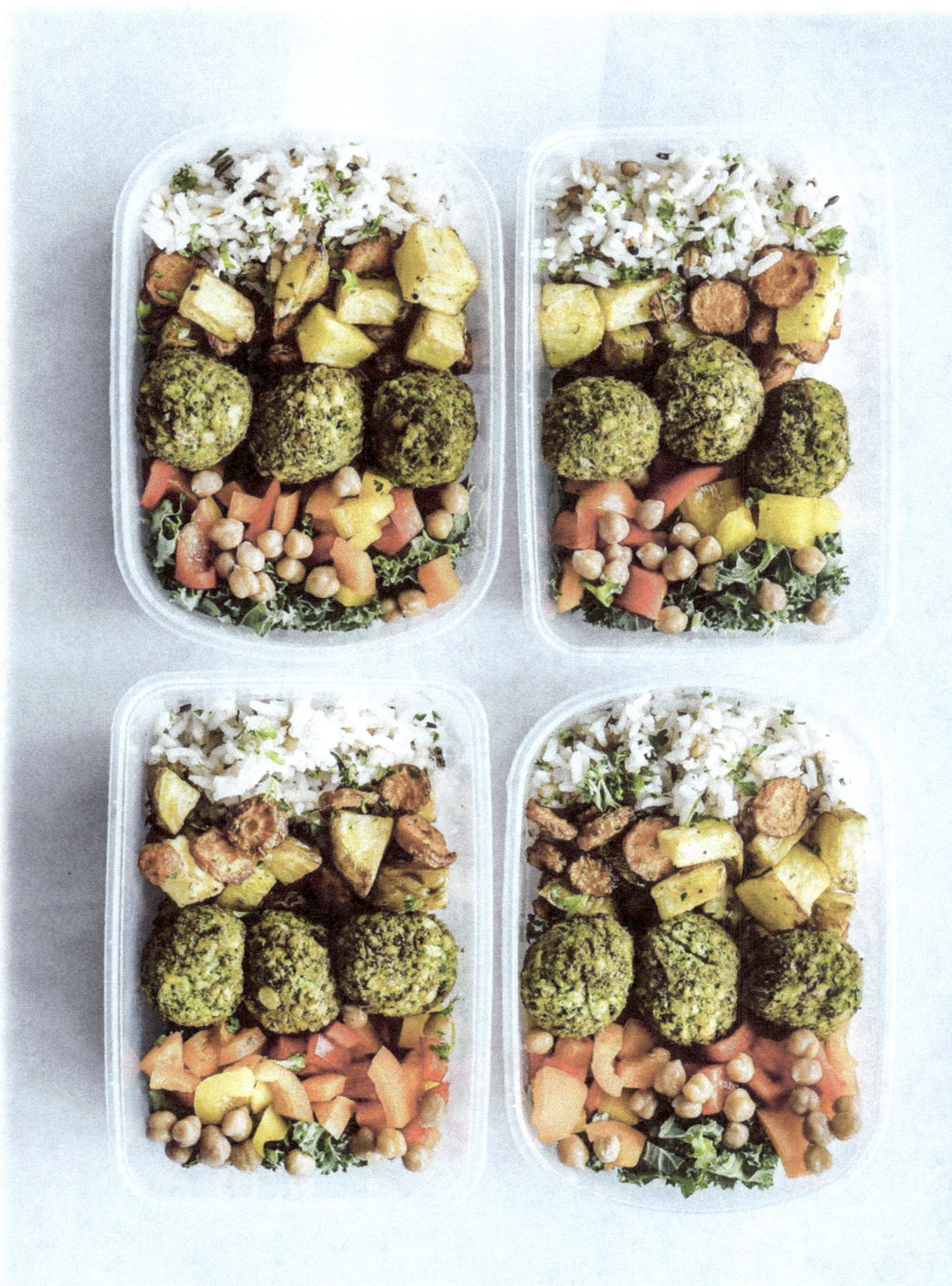

CONTENTS

Introduction

Understanding the DASH Diet

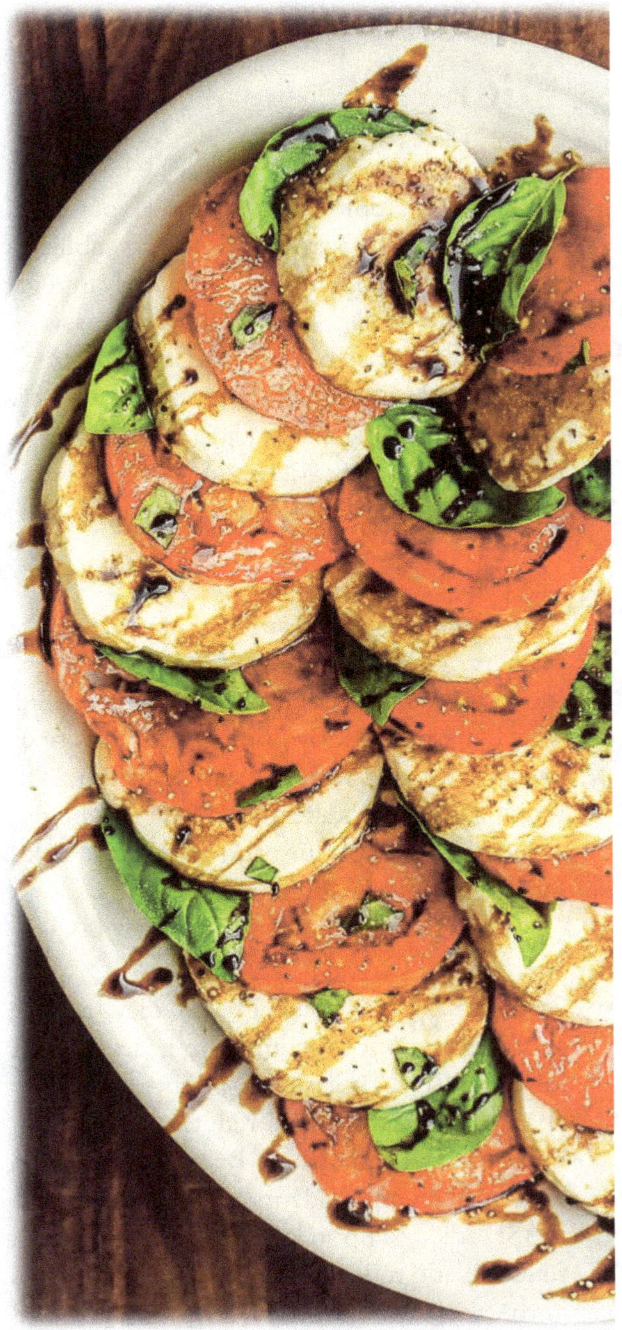

The Dietary Approaches to Stop Hypertension (DASH) diet is more than just a temporary eating plan; it's a lifestyle approach to healthy eating that has been shown to reduce blood pressure and enhance general well-being. The DASH diet was created by the National Heart, Lung, and Blood Institute (NHLBI) is backed by extensive scientific research and is recommended by healthcare professionals worldwide for its effectiveness in lowering the chance of stroke, heart disease, and other long-term illnesses.

Origins and Purpose

The DASH diet was initially created with the primary goal of lowering blood pressure, especially for individuals with hypertension (high blood pressure). However, its benefits extend beyond blood pressure management, as it promotes overall heart health and contributes to weight loss and improved overall well-being. The diet emphasizes the consumption of nutrient-rich foods while limiting sodium, saturated fats, and processed foods.

Key Principles

At its core, the DASH diet encourages the consumption of foods that are rich in essential nutrients, such as potassium, calcium, magnesium, and fiber, while minimizing the intake of sodium and unhealthy fats. It is characterized by its emphasis on whole foods, including fruits, vegetables, whole grains, lean proteins, and low-fat dairy products.

Food Groups and Servings

The DASH diet divides food into specific groups and recommends servings from each group based on a person's daily calorie needs. These food groups include:

- ❖ **Fruits**: Emphasizes a variety of fresh, frozen, or canned fruits without added sugars. Examples include apples, oranges, berries, and melons.
- ❖ **Vegetables**: Encourages a wide range of colorful vegetables, both raw and cooked, to maximize nutrient intake. Leafy greens, carrots, broccoli, and peppers are among the recommended choices.
- ❖ **Grains**: Prioritizes whole grains over refined grains, such as whole wheat bread, brown rice, oats, and quinoa. These provide fiber, vitamins, and minerals essential for heart health.
- ❖ **Protein**: Promotes lean sources of protein, such as poultry, fish, beans, lentils, tofu, and nuts. These options are lower in saturated fat and cholesterol compared to red meat and processed meats.
- ❖ **Dairy**: Recommends low-fat or fat-free dairy products, including milk, yogurt, and cheese, to meet calcium and vitamin D requirements while minimizing saturated fat intake.
- ❖ **Fats and Oils**: Encourages healthy fats, such as those found in olive oil, avocado, nuts, and seeds, while limiting saturated and trans fats found in butter, margarine, and processed foods.
- ❖ **Sweets and Added Sugars**: Advises moderation in consuming sweets and added sugars, including sugary beverages, desserts, and sweetened snacks.

Benefits of the DASH Diet

The Dietary Approaches to Stop Hypertension (DASH) diet is renowned for its ability to improve health outcomes, particularly in regard to cardiovascular health. Its emphasis on whole, nutrient-rich foods and its restriction of sodium and unhealthy fats contribute to a wide array of benefits beyond just blood pressure management. Let's delve into the extensive benefits of the DASH diet:

1. Blood Pressure Management: One of the primary aims of the DASH diet is to lower blood pressure levels, especially for individuals with hypertension. By prioritizing foods rich in potassium, magnesium, and calcium while limiting sodium intake, the DASH diet helps to regulate blood pressure and reduce the risk of hypertension-related complications.

2. Heart Health: The DASH diet has been shown to significantly improve heart health by lowering LDL cholesterol (often referred to as "bad" cholesterol) and reducing the risk of heart disease and stroke. By promoting a diet high in fiber, antioxidants, and healthy fats, the DASH diet supports optimal cardiovascular function and reduces the risk of plaque buildup in the arteries.

3. Weight Management: Following the DASH diet can aid in weight management and support healthy weight loss goals. Its emphasis on whole foods, such as fruits, vegetables, lean proteins, and whole grains, helps individuals feel satisfied while consuming fewer calories. Additionally, the diet discourages the consumption of high-calorie, processed foods, which can contribute to weight gain and obesity.

4. Diabetes Prevention and Management: The DASH diet's focus on balanced meals composed of complex carbohydrates, lean proteins, and healthy fats can help regulate blood sugar levels and improve insulin sensitivity. This makes it an effective dietary approach for preventing type 2 diabetes and managing blood sugar levels in individuals with diabetes.

5. Improved Nutrient Intake: By encouraging the consumption of a wide variety of nutrient-dense foods, the DASH diet ensures that individuals meet their daily requirements for essential vitamins, minerals, and antioxidants. This can lead to improved overall health, enhanced immune function, and better energy levels.

6. Reduced Risk of Chronic Diseases: Following the DASH diet has been associated with a decreased risk of developing chronic diseases beyond hypertension and heart disease. Studies have shown that adhering to the DASH diet can lower the risk of certain cancers, such as colorectal cancer, as well as reduce the incidence of osteoporosis, kidney stones, and other health conditions.

7. Long-Term Health and Well-Being: Embracing the principles of the DASH diet promotes a sustainable approach to healthy eating and lifestyle habits. By emphasizing whole, minimally processed foods and encouraging mindful eating practices, the DASH diet supports long-term health and well-being. Its flexible nature allows individuals to adapt the diet to their personal preferences and cultural traditions, making it easier to maintain over time.

The benefits of the DASH diet extend far beyond its ability to lower blood pressure. By promoting a balanced and nutritious eating pattern, the DASH diet improves heart health, supports weight management, reduces the risk of chronic diseases, and enhances overall well-being. Incorporating DASH-friendly foods into your daily meals can lead to significant improvements in health outcomes and contribute to a healthier, happier life.

Getting Started with the DASH Diet Cookbook

Embarking on a journey to embrace the principles of the DASH (Dietary Approaches to Stop Hypertension) diet is a significant step towards improving your overall health and well-being. The DASH diet emphasizes the consumption of nutrient-rich foods while limiting sodium, saturated fats, and processed foods, making it an effective dietary approach for reducing blood pressure and lowering the risk of heart disease and other chronic conditions. To help you get started on your DASH diet journey, here's a comprehensive guide to using the DASH Diet Cookbook:

1. Understanding the DASH Diet:
Before diving into the recipes, it's essential to familiarize yourself with the key principles of the DASH diet. Learn about the recommended food groups, serving sizes, and dietary guidelines that form the foundation of the DASH eating plan. Understanding why certain foods are emphasized while others are limited will help you make informed choices when selecting recipes from the cookbook.

2. Assessing Your Current Eating Habits:

Take some time to assess your current eating habits and identify areas where you can make improvements. Are you consuming enough fruits and vegetables each day? Are you mindful of your sodium intake? Are you incorporating whole grains and lean proteins into your meals? By identifying areas for improvement, you can set realistic goals for transitioning to a DASH-friendly diet.

3. Setting Realistic Goals:
Setting realistic and achievable goals is key to success when starting any new dietary regimen. Whether your goal is to lower your blood pressure, improve your heart health, or lose weight, establishing clear objectives will help you stay motivated and focused on your journey. Consider setting both short-term and long-term goals that align with the principles of the DASH diet.

4. Meal Planning and Preparation:
Meal planning and preparation are essential components of a successful DASH diet journey. Begin by browsing through the recipes in the DASH Diet Cookbook and selecting meals that appeal to you and align with your dietary goals. Create a weekly meal plan that includes a variety of DASH-friendly recipes for breakfast, lunch, dinner, and snacks. Make a shopping list of the ingredients you'll need and dedicate time each week to meal prep to ensure that healthy options are readily available.

5. Exploring the Cookbook:
The DASH Diet Cookbook contains a diverse range of recipes designed to make it easy and enjoyable to follow the DASH eating plan. From flavorful breakfast options and satisfying main dishes to nutritious snacks and desserts, there's something for everyone in the cookbook. Take the time to explore the different sections of the cookbook and experiment with new ingredients and flavors to keep your meals exciting and varied.

6. Incorporating DASH-Friendly Foods:
Focus on incorporating DASH-friendly foods into your meals, such as fruits, vegetables, whole grains, lean proteins, and low-fat dairy products. Experiment with different cooking methods and flavor combinations to create delicious and satisfying meals that align with the DASH diet principles. Be mindful of portion sizes and aim to fill your plate with a balance of nutrient-rich foods from all food groups.

7. Tracking Your Progress:
Keep track of your progress as you navigate your DASH diet journey. Monitor your blood pressure readings, weight, and other relevant health markers to gauge the effectiveness of the diet in achieving your goals. Pay attention to how you feel physically and emotionally as you adopt

healthier eating habits and make adjustments to your diet as needed.

Getting started with the DASH Diet Cookbook is an exciting opportunity to embrace a healthier way of eating and improve your overall health. By understanding the principles of the DASH diet, setting realistic goals, meal planning and preparation, exploring the cookbook, incorporating DASH-friendly foods, and tracking your progress, you'll be well-equipped to embark on a successful DASH diet journey. Remember to approach the process with patience, consistency, and a willingness to experiment with new foods and flavors.

Essential Ingredients and Kitchen Tools for the DASH Diet Cookbook

In order to fully embrace the principles of the DASH (Dietary Approaches to Stop Hypertension) diet and make the most of the recipes in the DASH Diet Cookbook, it's important to have a well-stocked kitchen and the necessary tools for preparing healthy and delicious meals. Here's a comprehensive guide to essential ingredients and kitchen tools for your DASH diet journey:

Essential Ingredients:

❖ **Fruits and Vegetables:** Fresh, frozen, or canned fruits and vegetables are foundational to the DASH diet. Stock up on a variety of colorful produce, including leafy greens, berries, citrus fruits, carrots, bell peppers, tomatoes, and more. Opt for fresh whenever possible, but frozen and canned options can be convenient and equally nutritious.

❖ **Whole Grains:** Whole grains provide fiber, vitamins, and minerals essential for heart health. Choose whole grain options such as brown rice, quinoa, oats, barley, whole wheat pasta, and whole grain bread. Incorporate these into your meals as a nutritious base or side dish.

❖ **Lean Proteins:** Lean proteins are an important component of the DASH diet. Opt for lean cuts of poultry (such as skinless chicken breast or turkey), fish (such as salmon or tilapia), beans, lentils, tofu, and legumes. These sources of protein are low in saturated fat and provide essential nutrients.

❖ **Low-Fat Dairy Products:** Low-fat or fat-free dairy products are rich in calcium and vitamin D, which are important for bone health. Include options such as skim milk, Greek yogurt, cottage cheese, and reduced-fat cheese in your diet.

❖ **Healthy Fats:** Incorporate healthy fats into your meals, such as olive oil, avocado, nuts, seeds, and fatty fish like salmon and mackerel. These fats provide essential fatty acids and can help promote heart health when consumed in moderation.

❖ **Herbs and Spices:** Herbs and spices add flavor to your dishes without the need for excess salt or sodium. Stock your pantry with a variety of herbs and spices, such as garlic, ginger, basil, oregano, cumin, turmeric, and cinnamon, to enhance the taste of your meals.

❖ **Low-Sodium Condiments and Flavorings:** Choose low-sodium versions of condiments and flavorings, such as reduced-sodium soy sauce, vinegar, lemon juice, and salsa, to season your meals without adding extra sodium.

Kitchen Tools:

❖ **Sharp Knives:** A set of sharp knives is essential for chopping, slicing, and dicing fruits, vegetables, and proteins with precision and ease.

❖ **Cutting Boards:** Invest in high-quality cutting boards to protect your countertops and provide a stable surface for food preparation. Consider having separate boards for raw meat, poultry, and produce to prevent cross-contamination.

❖ **Vegetable Peeler:** A vegetable peeler is useful for quickly and efficiently peeling fruits and vegetables, such as carrots, potatoes, and cucumbers.

❖ **Measuring Cups and Spoons:** Accurate measuring cups and spoons are essential for portion control and ensuring precise measurements of ingredients, especially when following recipes.

❖ **Mixing Bowls:** A set of mixing bowls in various sizes is handy for mixing ingredients, marinating meats, and storing leftovers.

❖ **Non-Stick Skillet and Saucepan:** Non-stick cookware makes cooking healthier meals with minimal added fats or oils easier. Invest in a quality non-stick skillet and saucepan for sautéing, frying, and simmering.

❖ **Baking Sheets and Pans:** Baking sheets and pans are versatile tools for roasting vegetables, baking proteins, and preparing healthy desserts. Look for non-stick options for easier cleanup.

❖ **Blender or Food Processor:** A blender or food processor is useful for making smoothies, pureeing soups, and creating homemade sauces and dressings.

❖ **Steamer Basket:** A steamer basket is a healthy cooking tool that allows you to steam vegetables while preserving their nutrients and natural flavors.

❖ **Food Storage Containers:** Invest in a set of food storage containers for storing leftovers, prepped ingredients, and meals for convenient grab-and-go options.

By stocking your kitchen with essential ingredients and having the right tools at your disposal, you'll be well-equipped to prepare delicious and nutritious meals that align with the principles of the DASH diet. Experiment with different flavors and ingredients to keep your meals exciting and satisfying as you embark on your DASH diet journey with the help of the DASH Diet Cookbook.

Tips for Success on the DASH Diet

Embracing the principles of the DASH (Dietary Approaches to Stop Hypertension) diet can lead to significant improvements in your health and well-being. Whether you're looking to lower your blood pressure, improve your heart health, or simply adopt a more nutritious eating pattern, these tips will help you succeed on your DASH diet journey:

1. Educate Yourself About the DASH Diet: Take the time to learn about the key principles of the DASH diet, including the recommended food groups, serving sizes, and dietary guidelines. Understanding the science behind the diet and its potential health benefits will help you stay motivated and committed to your goals.

2. Start Gradually: Transitioning to a new way of eating can be challenging, so start gradually by making small changes to your diet. Begin by incorporating more fruits, vegetables, and whole grains into your meals while gradually reducing your intake of sodium, saturated fats, and processed foods.

3. Focus on Whole, Nutrient-Rich Foods: Base your meals around whole, nutrient-rich foods such as fruits, vegetables, whole grains, lean proteins, and low-fat dairy products. These foods are rich in essential nutrients and fiber, which are important for heart health and overall well-being.

4. Plan Your Meals: Plan your meals ahead of time to ensure that you have healthy options available throughout the week. Create a weekly meal plan, make a shopping list, and dedicate time each week to meal prep. Having nutritious meals and snacks readily available will make it easier to stick to the DASH diet.

5. Experiment with Flavors and Ingredients: Explore new flavors and ingredients to keep your meals interesting and satisfying. Experiment with different herbs, spices, and cooking techniques to enhance the taste of your dishes without relying on excess salt or sodium.

6. Read Food Labels: Become familiar with reading food labels to identify high-sodium and high-fat foods that may not align with the DASH diet guidelines. Pay attention to serving sizes, sodium content, and ingredients lists when shopping for groceries.

7. Practice Portion Control: Pay attention to portion sizes and avoid overeating, even when consuming healthy foods. Use measuring cups, spoons, and kitchen scales to portion out your meals and snacks, especially when following recipes from the DASH Diet Cookbook.

8. Remain Hydrated: To promote general health and keep hydrated, sip lots of water throughout the day. Limit your intake of sugary beverages, caffeinated drinks, and alcohol, as these can contribute to dehydration and excess calorie consumption.

9. Be Mindful of Your Salt Intake: Reduce your intake of sodium by cooking at home more often and using fresh herbs, spices, and citrus juices to flavor your meals instead of salt. Reduce the amount of packaged and processed foods you eat because they are frequently heavy in salt.

10. Seek Support and Accountability: Enlist the support of friends, family members, or a registered dietitian who can provide encouragement and accountability as you navigate your DASH diet journey. Joining online forums or support groups can also connect you with like-minded individuals who are following similar dietary patterns.

11. Monitor Your Progress: Keep track of your progress by monitoring your blood pressure, weight, and other relevant health markers regularly. Celebrate your successes and use any setbacks as learning opportunities to adjust your approach and stay on track towards your goals.

12. Practice Self-Care: Prioritize self-care and stress management as part of your overall health and well-being. Engage in activities that help you relax and unwind, such as meditation, yoga, exercise, or spending time outdoors. Managing stress can have a positive impact on your physical and mental health.

By incorporating these tips into your daily routine, you'll set yourself up for success on the DASH diet. Remember that adopting a healthier lifestyle is a journey, and it's okay to take it one step at a time. With dedication, patience, and a positive mindset, you can achieve lasting improvements in your health and well-being with the help of the DASH Diet Cookbook.

1

Introduction to Breakfast Recipes

Introduction to Breakfast Recipes

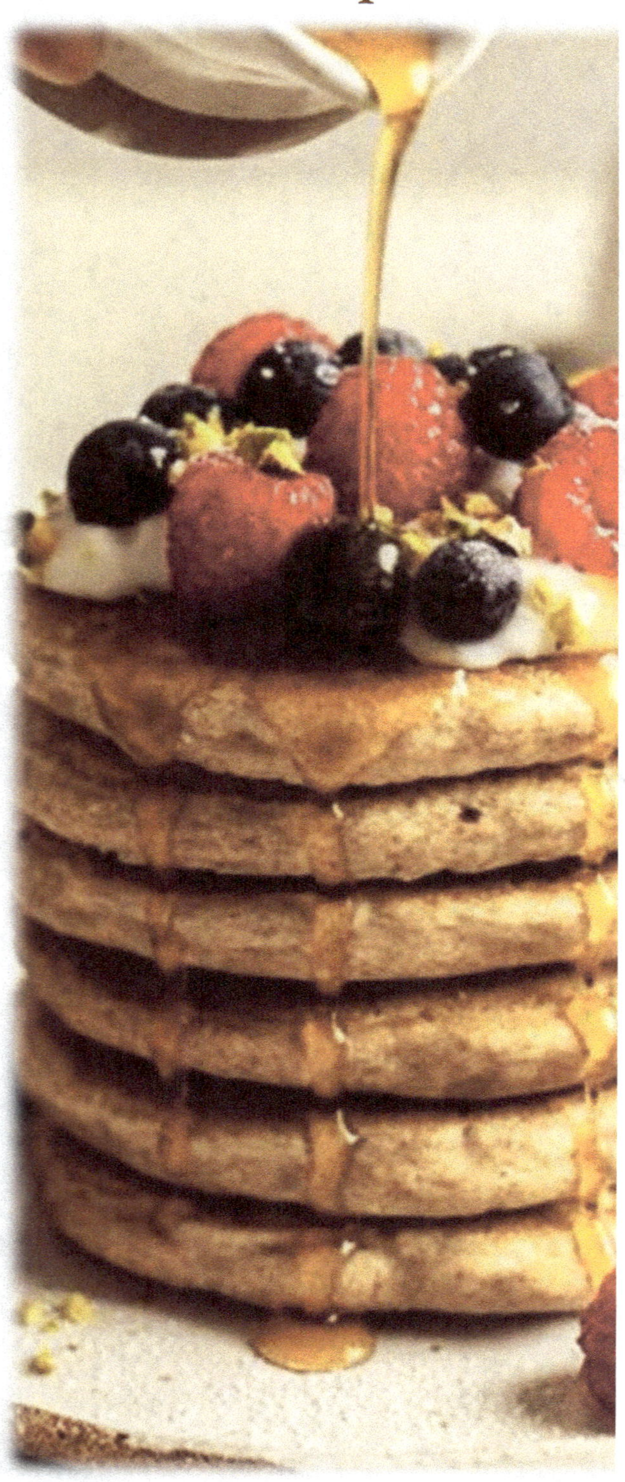

Breakfast is often referred to as the most important meal of the day, and with good reason. It sets the tone for your energy levels and appetite throughout the day. In the context of the DASH (Dietary Approaches to Stop Hypertension) diet, breakfast is an opportunity to kick‚start your day with nutrient-rich foods that support heart health and overall well-being.

The breakfast recipes featured in the DASH Diet Cookbook are designed to provide a delicious and satisfying start to your morning while adhering to the principles of the DASH diet. From hearty breakfast bowls packed with whole grains and fresh fruits to protein-packed omelettes and energizing smoothies, these recipes offer a variety of options to suit your tastes and dietary preferences.

By incorporating DASH-friendly breakfasts into your daily routine, you'll not only fuel your body with essential nutrients but also set yourself up for success in following a balanced and nutritious eating pattern throughout the day. Whether you prefer a quick and easy breakfast on-the-go or a leisurely brunch spread, the DASH Diet Cookbook has you covered with a selection of wholesome and delicious breakfast recipes to suit every palate.

Quinoa Breakfast Bowl

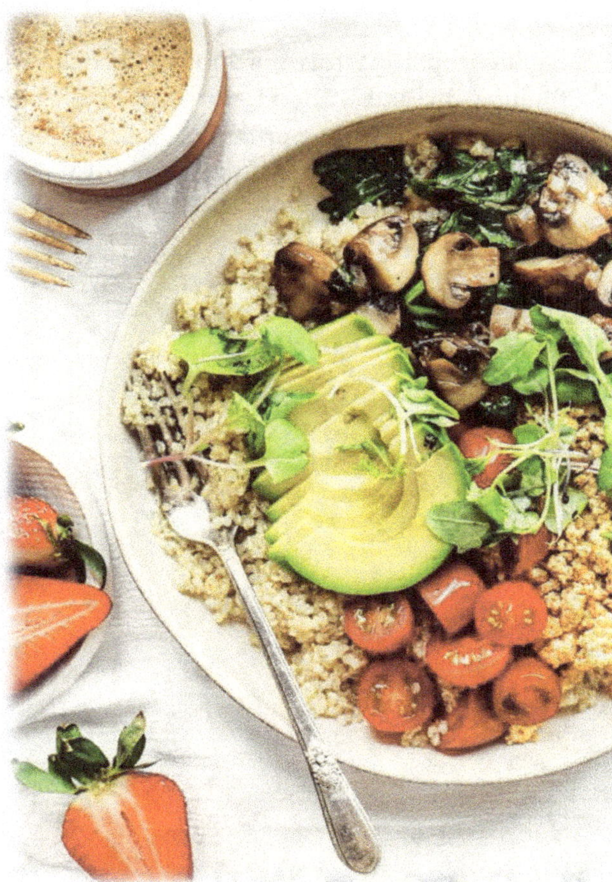

- ❖ **Preparation Time**: 5 minutes
- ❖ **Cooking Time**: 15 minutes
- ❖ **Serving Unit**: 1 bowl

Ingredients:

- ❖ 1/2 cup quinoa, rinsed
- ❖ 1 cup water or low-sodium vegetable broth
- ❖ 1/2 teaspoon ground cinnamon
- ❖ 1/4 teaspoon vanilla extract
- ❖ Half a cup of fresh berries, such raspberries, blueberries, or strawberries
- ❖ 1/4 cup chopped nuts or seeds (such as almonds, walnuts, or pumpkin seeds)
- ❖ 1 tablespoon honey or maple syrup (optional)
- ❖ Greek yogurt or low-fat milk, for serving (optional)

Procedures:

- ❖ In a small saucepan, combine the rinsed quinoa and water or vegetable broth. Bring to a boil over medium heat.
- ❖ Reduce the heat to low, cover, and simmer for 15 minutes, or until the quinoa is cooked and the liquid is absorbed.
- ❖ After turning off the heat, leave the pot covered for five minutes. Fluff the quinoa with a fork.
- ❖ Stir in the ground cinnamon and vanilla extract until well combined.
- ❖ Transfer the cooked quinoa to a serving bowl.
- ❖ Top the quinoa with fresh berries, chopped nuts or seeds, and a drizzle of honey or maple syrup, if desired.
- ❖ Serve the quinoa breakfast bowl with a dollop of Greek yogurt or a splash of low-fat milk, if desired.

Nutritional Values (per serving):

- ❖ **Calories**: 350
- ❖ **Protein**: 12g
- ❖ **Carbohydrates**: 50g
- ❖ **Dietary** Fiber: 8g
- ❖ **Sugars**: 12g
- ❖ **Fat**: 12g
- ❖ **Saturated** Fat: 1g
- ❖ **Cholesterol**: 0mg
- ❖ **Sodium**: 10mg

* **Potassium**: 480mg
* **Calcium**: 80mg
* **Iron**: 3mg

Cooking Tips:

* Rinse the quinoa thoroughly before cooking to remove any bitter coating called saponin.
* Use low-sodium vegetable broth instead of water for added flavor.
* Customize your breakfast bowl with your favorite fruits, nuts, seeds, and sweeteners.
* Make a batch of quinoa ahead of time and store it in the refrigerator for quick and easy breakfasts throughout the week.

Health Benefits:

* **Rich in Protein:** Quinoa is a complete protein, containing all nine essential amino acids, making it an excellent choice for vegetarians and vegans.
* **High in Fiber:** Quinoa is a good source of dietary fiber, which helps promote digestive health, regulate blood sugar levels, and keep you feeling full and satisfied.
* **Packed with Nutrients:** Quinoa is rich in vitamins, minerals, and antioxidants, including magnesium, phosphorus, manganese, and folate, which are essential for overall health and well-being.
* **Heart-Healthy:** Quinoa is low in saturated fat and cholesterol-free, making it a heart-healthy choice that can help lower the risk of heart disease and improve cardiovascular health.

* **Gluten-Free:** Quinoa is naturally gluten-free, making it suitable for individuals with celiac disease or gluten sensitivity.

By incorporating this nutritious and delicious Quinoa Breakfast Bowl into your morning routine, you'll start your day on a healthy and satisfying note, setting the stage for a day filled with energy and vitality.

Veggie-Packed Omelette

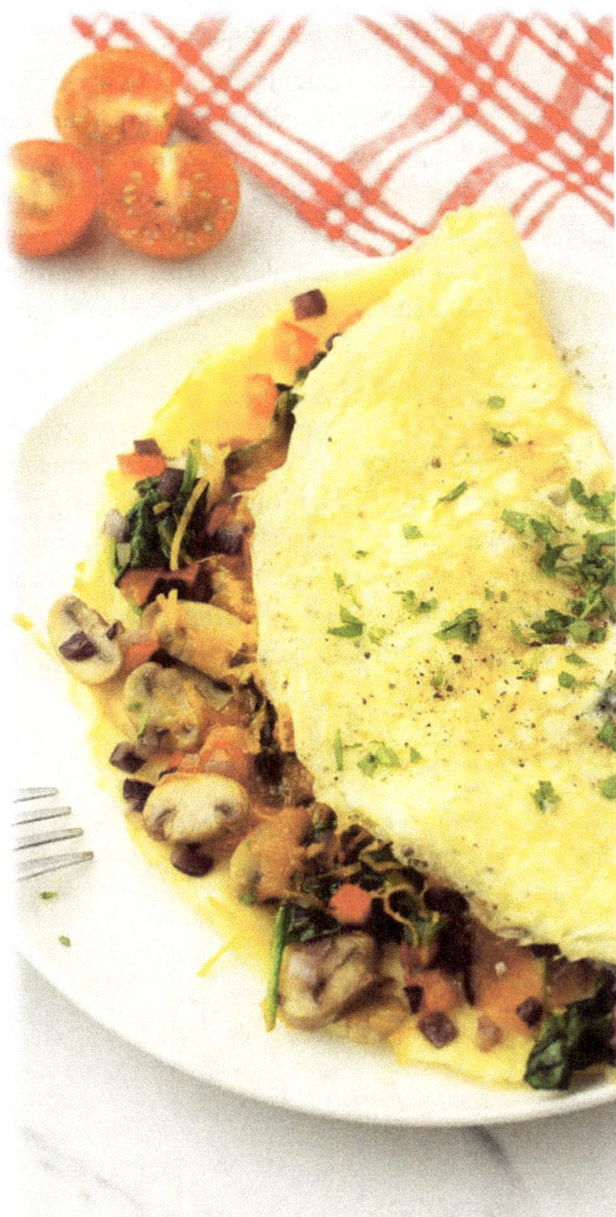

Ingredients:

- 2 large eggs
- 1/4 cup chopped mixed vegetables (such as bell peppers, onions, tomatoes, spinach, mushrooms, or broccoli)
- 1 tablespoon of freshly chopped herbs, such parsley, basil, or chives.
- 1 tablespoon cooking spray or olive oil
- Salt and pepper, to taste
- 1/4 cup shredded cheese (such as cheddar, mozzarella, or feta), optional

Procedures:

- In a small bowl, beat the eggs until well mixed. Season with salt and pepper, if desired.
- Heat the olive oil or cooking spray in a non-stick skillet over medium heat.
- Add the chopped vegetables to the skillet and sauté for 2-3 minutes, or until they are tender.
- Pour the beaten eggs over the sautéed vegetables, tilting the skillet to distribute the eggs evenly.
- Cook the omelette for 2-3 minutes, or until the edges begin to set and the bottom is lightly golden brown.
- Sprinkle the chopped fresh herbs and shredded cheese (if using) evenly over one half of the omelette.
- Using a spatula, carefully fold the other half of the omelette over the filling to form a half-moon shape.
- Cook for an additional 1-2 minutes, or until the cheese is melted and the eggs are cooked through.
- Transfer the omelette to a platter and start serving right away.

Preparation Time: 10 minutes

Cooking Time: 10 minutes

Serving Unit: 1 omelette

Nutritional Values (per serving without cheese):

- ❖ **Calories**: 150
- ❖ **Protein**: 12g
- ❖ **Carbohydrates**: 4g
- ❖ **Dietary Fiber**: 1g
- ❖ **Sugars**: 2g
- ❖ **Fat**: 10g
- ❖ **Saturated Fat**: 2g
- ❖ **Cholesterol**: 370mg
- ❖ **Sodium**: 130mg
- ❖ **Potassium**: 200mg
- ❖ **Calcium**: 50mg
- ❖ **Iron**: 1mg

Cooking Tips:

- ❖ Use a non-stick skillet to prevent the omelette from sticking and facilitate flipping.
- ❖ Chop the vegetables into small, uniform pieces for even cooking and distribution throughout the omelette.
- ❖ Customize the omelette with your favorite vegetables and herbs for added flavor and nutritional variety.
- ❖ Be mindful not to overfill the omelette, as it may become difficult to fold and flip.

Health Benefits:

- ❖ **High in Protein:** Eggs are a rich source of high-quality protein, which is essential for muscle repair and growth, as well as satiety.
- ❖ **Loaded with Nutrients:** Eggs are packed with essential vitamins and minerals, including vitamin D, vitamin B12, selenium, and choline, which support overall health and well-being.
- ❖ **Rich in Vegetables:** This omelette is packed with nutrient-rich vegetables, which provide vitamins, minerals, fiber, and antioxidants that promote optimal health and reduce the risk of chronic diseases.
- ❖ **Low in Calories:** This veggie-packed omelette is low in calories but high in volume, making it a satisfying and nutritious breakfast option that can support weight management goals.
- ❖ **Versatile and Customizable:** You can customize this omelette with your favorite vegetables, herbs, and cheeses to suit your taste preferences and dietary needs.

By incorporating this Veggie-Packed Omelette into your breakfast routine, you'll enjoy a delicious and nutritious meal that provides essential nutrients, supports satiety, and sets the stage for a day filled with energy and vitality.

Berry Blast Smoothie

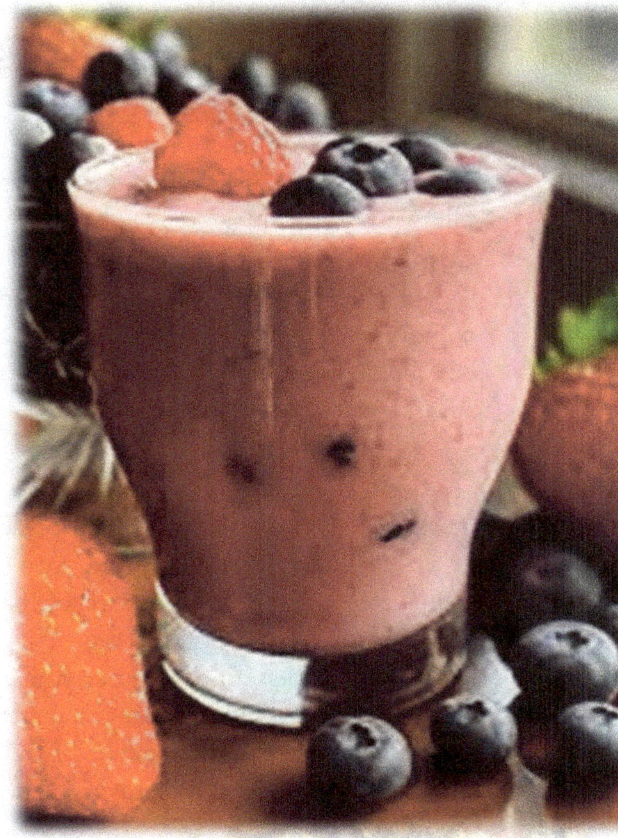

Preparation Time: 5 minutes

Cooking Time: 0 minutes

Serving Unit: 1 smoothie

Ingredients:

- ❖ 1/2 cup mixed berries (such as strawberries, blueberries, raspberries, or blackberries), fresh or frozen
- ❖ 1/2 banana, fresh or frozen
- ❖ 1/2 cup dairy-free yogurt or plain Greek yogurt
- ❖ 1/2 cup unsweetened almond milk or any milk of your choice
- ❖ 1 tablespoon honey or maple syrup (optional)
- ❖ 1/2 teaspoon vanilla extract
- ❖ Ice cubes (optional)

Procedures:

- ❖ Place the mixed berries, banana, Greek yogurt, almond milk, honey or maple syrup (if using), and vanilla extract in a blender.
- ❖ If you would want the smoothie to be thicker and colder, add a few ice cubes to the blender.
- ❖ Blend on high speed until smooth and creamy, scraping down the sides of the blender as needed to ensure all ingredients are well incorporated.
- ❖ Taste the smoothie and adjust sweetness as needed by adding more honey or maple syrup, if desired.
- ❖ Once the desired consistency and sweetness are achieved, pour the Berry Blast Smoothie into a glass and serve immediately.

Nutritional Values (per serving):

- ❖ **Calories:** 180
- ❖ **Protein:** 15g
- ❖ **Carbohydrates:** 30g
- ❖ **Dietary Fiber:** 5g
- ❖ **Sugars:** 20g
- ❖ **Fat:** 2g
- ❖ **Saturated Fat:** 0g
- ❖ **Cholesterol:** 0mg
- ❖ **Sodium:** 80mg
- ❖ **Potassium:** 380mg
- ❖ **Calcium:** 200mg
- ❖ **Iron:** 1mg

Cooking Tips:

* Use a combination of fresh and frozen berries for the perfect balance of flavor and texture. The smoothie will be cooler and thicker with the addition of frozen berries.
* Freeze leftover ripe bananas for later use in smoothies. Frozen bananas add creaminess and natural sweetness to smoothies without the need for additional sweeteners.
* Customize the smoothie with your favorite add-ins, such as spinach, kale, protein powder, or nut butter, to boost its nutritional content and make it more filling.
* Adjust the consistency of the smoothie by adding more or less liquid (almond milk or yogurt) to achieve your desired thickness.

Health Benefits:

* **Rich in Antioxidants: Berries** are packed with antioxidants, such as anthocyanins and flavonoids, which help fight inflammation, protect against oxidative stress, and reduce the risk of chronic diseases, including heart disease and cancer.
* **Excellent Source of Vitamins and Minerals:** Berries are rich in essential vitamins and minerals, including vitamin C, vitamin K, manganese, and potassium, which support immune function, bone health, and electrolyte balance.
* **High in Fiber:** Berries are high in dietary fiber, which promotes digestive health, regulates blood sugar levels, and supports weight management by promoting feelings of fullness and reducing hunger cravings.
* **Protein-Packed:** Greek yogurt is a rich source of high-quality protein, which is essential for muscle repair and growth, as well as satiety. Adding Greek yogurt to the smoothie increases its protein content and makes it more filling and satisfying.
* **Low in Added Sugars:** This smoothie is naturally sweetened with fruit and contains no added sugars, making it a healthier alternative to store-bought smoothies and sugary beverages.

By incorporating this Berry Blast Smoothie into your breakfast or snack routine, you'll enjoy a delicious and nutritious beverage that provides a burst of flavor, essential nutrients, and numerous health benefits. Whether you're looking for a quick and convenient breakfast option or a refreshing post-workout snack, this smoothie is sure to satisfy your cravings and fuel your body with goodness.

Whole Wheat Pancakes with Fresh Fruit

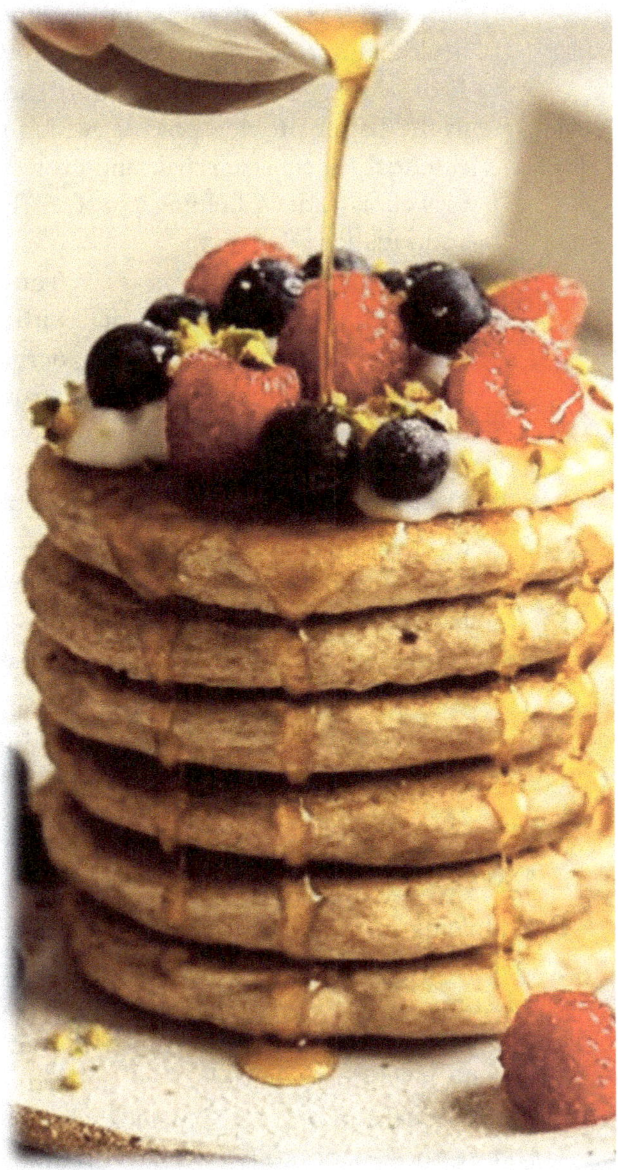

- ❖ **Preparation Time:** 10 minutes
- ❖ **Cooking Time:** 15 minutes
- ❖ **Serving Unit:** 2 pancakes

Ingredients:

- ❖ 1 cup whole wheat flour
- ❖ 1 tablespoon sugar or your preferred sweetness
- ❖ 1 teaspoon baking powder
- ❖ 1/2 teaspoon baking soda
- ❖ 1/4 teaspoon salt
- ❖ 1 cup buttermilk or plain Greek yogurt mixed with milk
- ❖ 1 large egg
- ❖ 2 tablespoons unsalted butter, melted
- ❖ 1 teaspoon vanilla extract
- ❖ Fresh fruit (such as berries, sliced bananas, or diced apples), for topping
- ❖ Maple syrup or honey, for drizzling

Procedures:

- ❖ In a large mixing bowl, whisk together the whole wheat flour, sugar, baking powder, baking soda, and salt until well combined.
- ❖ In a separate bowl, whisk together the buttermilk (or yogurt and milk mixture), egg, melted butter, and vanilla extract until smooth.
- ❖ After adding the wet components to the dry ingredients, mix just until incorporated. A few lumps are OK; take care not to overmix.
- ❖ A nonstick skillet or griddle should be heated to medium heat. Lightly grease the skillet with cooking spray or a small amount of butter.
- ❖ For each pancake, add around 1/4 cup of batter to the skillet. Cook for 2-3 minutes, or until bubbles form on the surface and the edges begin to look set.
- ❖ Flip the pancakes and cook for an additional 1-2 minutes, or until golden brown and cooked through.

❖ Transfer the cooked pancakes to a plate and repeat with the remaining batter, greasing the skillet as needed.
❖ Serve the whole wheat pancakes topped with fresh fruit and a drizzle of maple syrup or honey.

Nutritional Values (per serving, without toppings):

❖ **Calories**: 200
❖ **Protein**: 7g
❖ **Carbohydrates**: 30g
❖ **Dietary Fiber**: 4g
❖ **Sugars**: 5g
❖ **Fat**: 6g
❖ **Saturated** Fat: 3g
❖ **Cholesterol**: 60mg
❖ **Sodium**: 400mg
❖ **Potassium**: 200mg
❖ **Calcium**: 100mg
❖ **Iron**: 2mg

Cooking Tips:

❖ To keep pancakes warm while cooking the remaining batches, place them on a baking sheet in a preheated oven set to 200°F (93°C).
❖ Use a measuring cup or ladle to portion out the pancake batter for consistent pancake sizes.
❖ Customize the pancakes by adding extras such as chocolate chips, nuts, or spices like cinnamon or nutmeg to the batter for added flavor and texture.
❖ For fluffier pancakes, avoid overmixing the batter and let it rest for a few minutes before cooking to allow the baking powder and baking soda to activate.

Health Benefits:

❖ **Whole Grains:** Whole wheat flour used in these pancakes is rich in fiber, vitamins, and minerals compared to refined flour, promoting digestive health and providing sustained energy.
❖ **Protein:** Eggs and Greek yogurt used in the batter provide protein, which is essential for muscle repair and growth, as well as satiety, helping you feel full and satisfied.
❖ **Low in Added Sugars:** These pancakes are lightly sweetened with a small amount of sugar and derive additional sweetness from fresh fruit, making them a healthier alternative to traditional pancakes loaded with syrup.
❖ **Heart-Healthy Fats:** Butter used in moderation provides a small amount of heart-healthy fats, while also adding flavor and moisture to the pancakes.
❖ **Nutrient-Dense Toppings:** Fresh fruit toppings add natural sweetness, fiber, vitamins, and antioxidants to the pancakes, enhancing their nutritional value and flavor.

By indulging in these Whole Wheat Pancakes with Fresh Fruit, you'll enjoy a delicious and wholesome breakfast that satisfies your taste buds while providing essential nutrients and numerous health benefits. Whether enjoyed as a leisurely weekend brunch or a quick weekday breakfast, these pancakes are sure to become a family favorite.

2

Introduction to Lunch Recipes

Introduction to Lunch Recipes

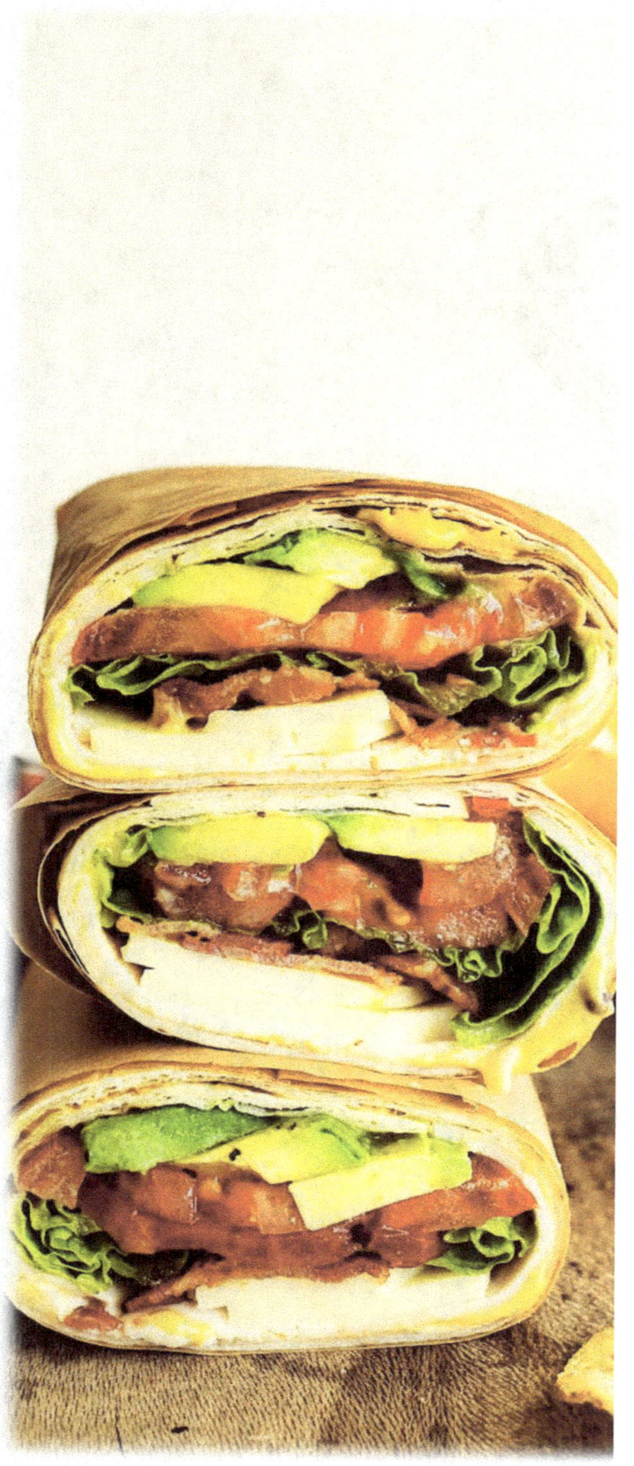

Lunch is an essential meal that provides the opportunity to refuel and recharge your body midday. In the context of the DASH (Dietary Approaches to Stop Hypertension) diet, lunch serves as an important opportunity to incorporate nutrient-rich foods that support heart health and overall well-being.

The lunch recipes featured in the DASH Diet Cookbook are designed to be flavorful, satisfying, and easy to prepare, making them perfect for busy weekdays or leisurely weekends. From vibrant salads and hearty soups to wholesome sandwiches and nourishing bowls, these recipes offer a variety of options to suit your tastes and dietary preferences.

By incorporating DASH-friendly lunch recipes into your meal planning, you'll not only nourish your body with essential nutrients but also enjoy delicious and satisfying meals that contribute to your overall health and wellness. Whether you're looking for a quick and convenient lunch option or a leisurely meal to enjoy with family and friends, the DASH Diet Cookbook has you covered with a selection of wholesome and nutritious lunch recipes to suit every palate.

Mediterranean Chickpea Salad

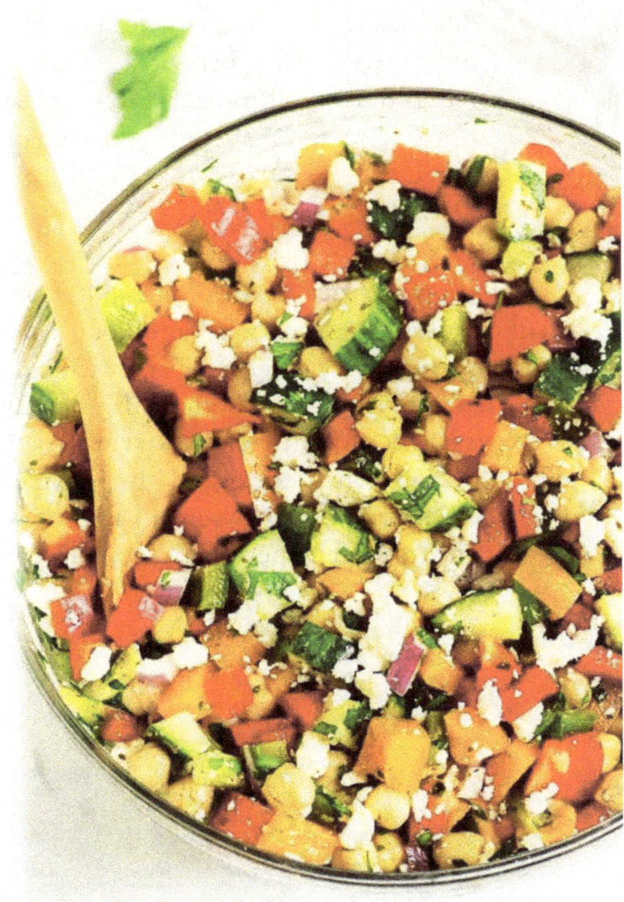

Ingredients:

- ❖ 1 can (15 ounces) of washed and drained garbanzo beans, or chickpeas
- ❖ 1 cup cherry tomatoes, halved
- ❖ 1/2 cucumber, diced
- ❖ 1/4 red onion, thinly sliced
- ❖ 1/4 cup Kalamata olives, pitted and halved
- ❖ 1/4 cup crumbled feta cheese
- ❖ 2 tablespoons chopped fresh parsley
- ❖ 2 tablespoons extra virgin olive oil
- ❖ 1 tablespoon lemon juice
- ❖ 1 teaspoon dried oregano
- ❖ Salt and pepper, to taste

Procedures:

- ❖ In a large mixing bowl, combine the chickpeas, cherry tomatoes, cucumber, red onion, Kalamata olives, feta cheese, and chopped fresh parsley.
- ❖ To create the dressing, combine the dried oregano, lemon juice, extra virgin olive oil, salt, and pepper in a small dish.
- ❖ After adding the dressing to the chickpea mixture, toss until well mixed.
- ❖ Taste and add more salt, pepper, or lemon juice to suit your taste.
- ❖ Serve the Mediterranean Chickpea Salad immediately, or refrigerate for at least 30 minutes to allow the flavors to meld before serving.

Nutritional Values (per serving):

- ❖ **Calories**: 350
- ❖ **Protein**: 12g
- ❖ **Carbohydrates**: 30g
- ❖ **Dietary Fiber**: 8g
- ❖ **Sugars**: 5g

- ❖ **Preparation Time**: 15 minutes
- ❖ **Cooking Time**: 0 minutes
- ❖ **Serving Unit**: 1 bowl

- ❖ **Fat**: 20g
- ❖ **Saturated Fat**: 4g
- ❖ **Cholesterol**: 10mg
- ❖ **Sodium**: 550mg
- ❖ **Potassium**: 450mg
- ❖ **Calcium**: 150mg
- ❖ **Iron**: 3mg

Cooking Tips:

- ❖ For best results, use canned chickpeas that have been drained and rinsed thoroughly to remove excess sodium and starch.
- ❖ Customize the salad by adding additional vegetables such as bell peppers, artichoke hearts, or avocado for added flavor and nutrition.
- ❖ Crumble the feta cheese just before serving to preserve its texture and prevent it from becoming too soggy.
- ❖ Make the dressing ahead of time and store it separately from the salad ingredients until ready to serve to prevent the salad from becoming too soggy.

Health Benefits:

- ❖ Rich in Protein and Fiber: Chickpeas are a good source of plant-based protein and dietary fiber, which promote satiety, regulate blood sugar levels, and support digestive health.
- ❖ Heart-Healthy Fats: Extra virgin olive oil used in the dressing provides heart-healthy monounsaturated fats, which help reduce inflammation and improve cholesterol levels.
- ❖ Loaded with Vitamins and Minerals: The variety of vegetables in this salad provide essential vitamins and minerals, including vitamin C, vitamin K, potassium, and antioxidants, which support immune function, bone health, and overall well-being.
- ❖ Low in Saturated Fat: This salad is low in saturated fat and cholesterol, making it a heart-healthy option that can help lower the risk of heart disease and improve cardiovascular health.
- ❖ Mediterranean Diet Benefits: This salad is inspired by the Mediterranean diet, which has been associated with numerous health benefits, including reduced risk of chronic diseases such as heart disease, diabetes, and certain cancers.

By incorporating this flavorful and nutritious Mediterranean Chickpea Salad into your lunch rotation, you'll enjoy a delicious and satisfying meal that nourishes your body with essential nutrients and contributes to your overall health and well-being. Whether enjoyed on its own or as a side dish, this salad is sure to become a favorite in your meal repertoire.

Turkey and Avocado Wrap

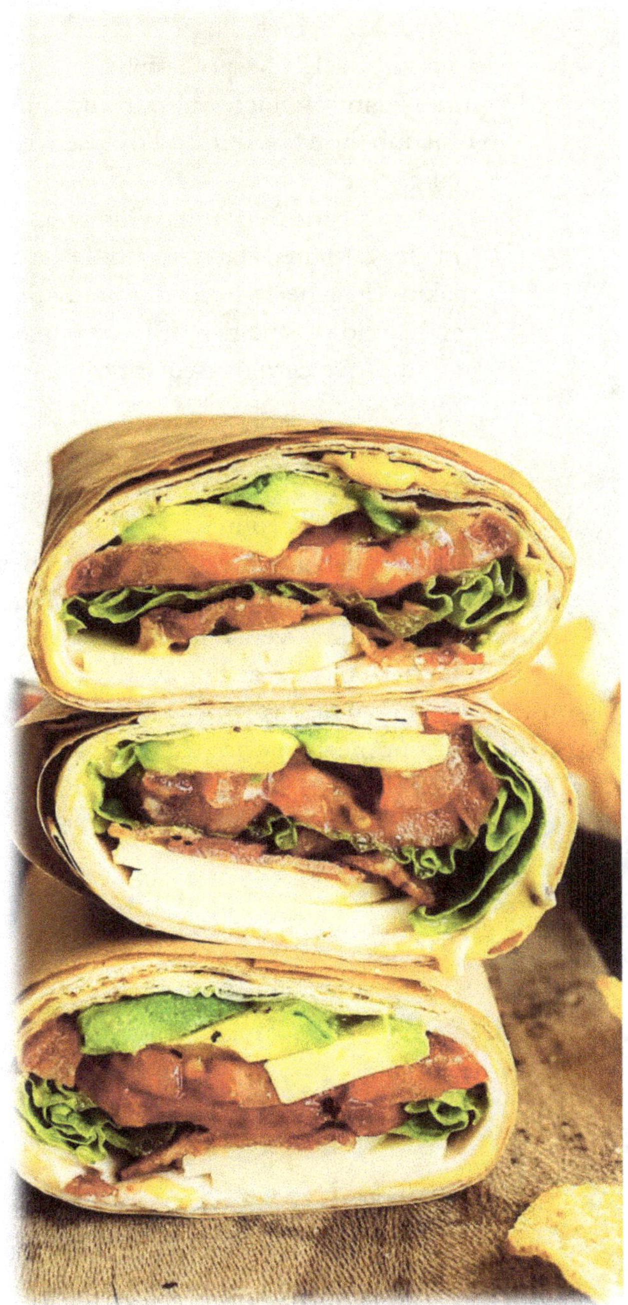

Ingredients:

- ❖ 1 whole wheat or multigrain tortilla wrap
- ❖ 3 ounces cooked turkey breast, sliced
- ❖ 1/4 avocado, sliced
- ❖ 1/4 cup shredded lettuce
- ❖ 2 slices tomato
- ❖ 2 slices cucumber
- ❖ 1 tablespoon hummus or mustard
- ❖ Salt and pepper, to taste

Procedures:

- ❖ Spoon the tortilla wrapper onto a sanitized surface.
- ❖ Spread the hummus or mustard evenly over the center of the tortilla.
- ❖ Layer the sliced turkey breast, avocado, shredded lettuce, tomato slices, and cucumber slices over the hummus or mustard.
- ❖ Season with salt and pepper, to taste.
- ❖ To construct a wrap, fold in the tortilla's sides and roll it firmly from the bottom.
- ❖ Slice the wrap in half diagonally, if desired, and serve immediately.

Nutritional Values (per serving):

- ❖ **Calories:** 300
- ❖ **Protein:** 20g
- ❖ **Carbohydrates:** 25g
- ❖ **Dietary Fiber:** 7g
- ❖ **Sugars:** 2g
- ❖ **Fat:** 15g
- ❖ **Saturated Fat:** 2g
- ❖ **Cholesterol:** 30mg

- ❖ **Preparation Time:** 10 minutes
- ❖ **Cooking Time:** 0 minutes
- ❖ **Serving Unit:** 1 wrap

- ❖ **Sodium**: 400mg
- ❖ **Potassium**: 450mg
- ❖ **Calcium**: 50mg
- ❖ **Iron**: 2mg

Cooking Tips:

- ❖ Use leftover cooked turkey breast or store-bought sliced turkey for convenience.
- ❖ Choose whole wheat or multigrain tortilla wraps for added fiber and nutrients.
- ❖ To prevent the wrap from becoming soggy, layer the ingredients evenly and avoid overfilling.
- ❖ Customize the wrap with additional vegetables, such as bell peppers, spinach, or red onion, for added flavor and nutrition.
- ❖ Secure the wrap with toothpicks or wrap it in parchment paper or aluminum foil for easy transport and eating on-the-go.

Health Benefits:

- ❖ **Lean Protein:** Turkey breast is a lean source of protein, which is essential for muscle repair and growth, as well as satiety, helping you feel full and satisfied.
- ❖ **Healthy Fats:** Avocado provides heart-healthy monounsaturated fats, which help reduce inflammation and improve cholesterol levels.
- ❖ **Fiber-Rich:** Whole wheat tortilla wraps and vegetables provide dietary fiber, which promotes digestive health, regulates blood sugar levels, and supports weight management by promoting feelings of fullness and reducing hunger cravings.
- ❖ **Nutrient-Dense:** This wrap is packed with essential vitamins and minerals from the turkey, avocado, and vegetables, including vitamin C, vitamin K, potassium, and antioxidants, which support immune function, bone health, and overall well-being.
- ❖ **Low in Saturated Fat:** This wrap is low in saturated fat and cholesterol, making it a heart-healthy option that can help lower the risk of heart disease and improve cardiovascular health.

By incorporating this Turkey and Avocado Wrap into your lunch routine, you'll enjoy a delicious and satisfying meal that nourishes your body with essential nutrients and contributes to your overall health and well-being. Whether enjoyed at home, at work, or on-the-go, this wrap is sure to become a favorite in your meal repertoire.

Zucchini Noodles with Pesto

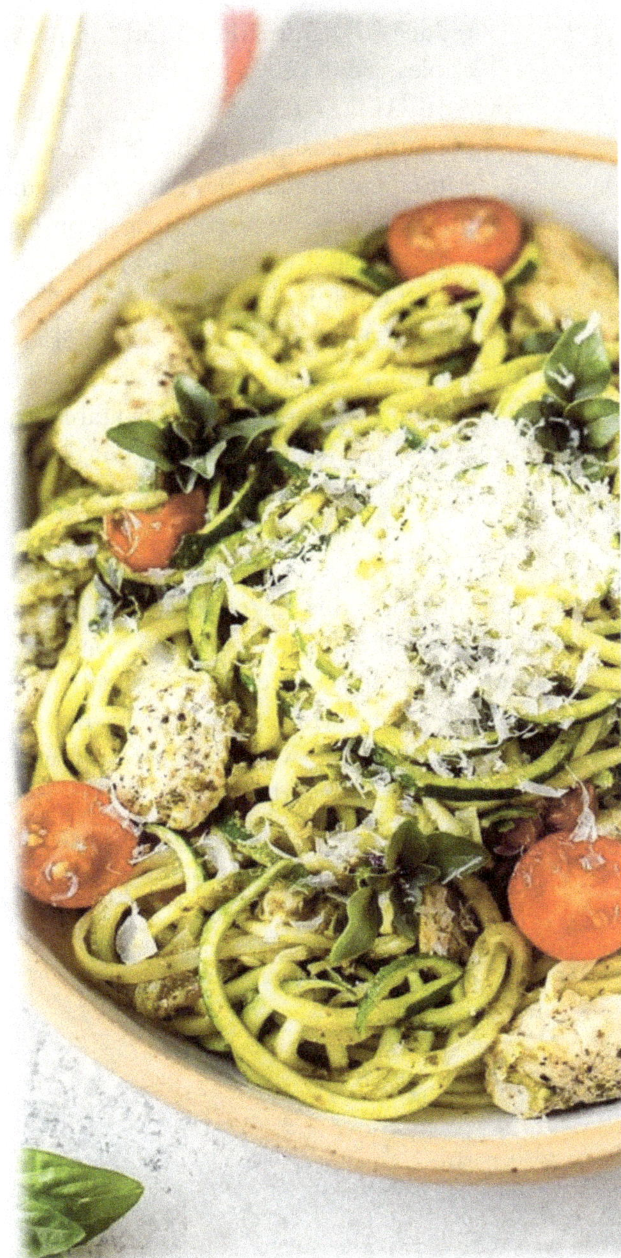

Ingredients:

- ❖ 2 medium zucchinis, spiralized into noodles
- ❖ 1/4 cup homemade or store-bought pesto sauce
- ❖ 1 tablespoon olive oil
- ❖ 2 cloves garlic, minced
- ❖ Salt and pepper, to taste
- ❖ Grated Parmesan cheese, for garnish (optional)
- ❖ Fresh basil leaves, for garnish (optional)

Procedures:

- ❖ In a large skillet set over medium heat, warm up the olive oil.
- ❖ Add minced garlic to the skillet and sauté for 1-2 minutes, or until fragrant.
- ❖ Add zucchini noodles to the skillet and toss to coat in the garlic-infused olive oil.
- ❖ Cook the zucchini noodles for 3-4 minutes, stirring occasionally, or until they are tender but still slightly crisp.
- ❖ Remove the skillet from heat and add pesto sauce to the zucchini noodles, tossing until they are evenly coated.
- ❖ Season with salt and pepper to taste.
- ❖ Transfer the zucchini noodles with pesto to a serving plate.
- ❖ If preferred, garnish with freshly chopped basil leaves and grated Parmesan cheese.
- ❖ Serve immediately, while hot.

- ❖ **Preparation Time:** 15 minutes
- ❖ **Cooking Time:** 10 minutes
- ❖ **Serving Unit:** 1 plate

Nutritional Values (per serving):

- ❖ **Calories:** 200
- ❖ **Protein:** 5g
- ❖ **Carbohydrates:** 10g

- ❖ **Dietary Fiber**: 3g
- ❖ **Sugars**: 5g
- ❖ **Fat**: 15g
- ❖ **Saturated Fat**: 3g
- ❖ **Cholesterol**: 5mg
- ❖ **Sodium**: 300mg
- ❖ **Potassium**: 500mg
- ❖ **Calcium**: 100mg
- ❖ **Iron**: 2mg

Cooking Tips:

- ❖ Use a spiralizer to create uniform zucchini noodles for best results.
- ❖ Be careful not to overcook the zucchini noodles, as they can become mushy and lose their texture.
- ❖ If you don't have a spiralizer, you can use a vegetable peeler to create long, thin strips of zucchini, similar to fettuccine noodles.
- ❖ Customize the pesto sauce by adding additional ingredients such as pine nuts, almonds, or spinach for added flavor and nutrition.
- ❖ Make extra pesto sauce and store it in an airtight container in the refrigerator for up to a week, or freeze it for longer storage.

Health Benefits:

- ❖ **Low in Calories and Carbohydrates:** Zucchini noodles are a low-calorie and low-carb alternative to traditional pasta, making them suitable for those watching their calorie and carbohydrate intake.
- ❖ **Rich in Vitamins and Minerals:** Zucchini is rich in essential vitamins and minerals, including vitamin C, vitamin K, potassium, and manganese, which support immune function, bone health, and electrolyte balance.
- ❖ **Heart-Healthy Fats:** Olive oil used in the recipe provides heart-healthy monounsaturated fats, which help reduce inflammation and improve cholesterol levels.
- ❖ **Antioxidant-Rich:** Pesto sauce contains basil, which is rich in antioxidants such as flavonoids and polyphenols, which help protect against oxidative stress and reduce the risk of chronic diseases.
- ❖ **Gluten-Free and Paleo-Friendly:** Zucchini noodles with pesto are naturally gluten-free and suitable for individuals following a paleo or gluten-free diet.

By incorporating this flavorful and nutritious Zucchini Noodles with Pesto into your meal rotation, you'll enjoy a delicious and satisfying dish that's packed with essential nutrients and contributes to your overall health and well-being. Whether enjoyed as a light lunch or a flavorful side dish, this recipe is sure to become a favorite in your culinary repertoire.

3

Introduction to Dinner Recipes

Introduction to Dinner Recipes

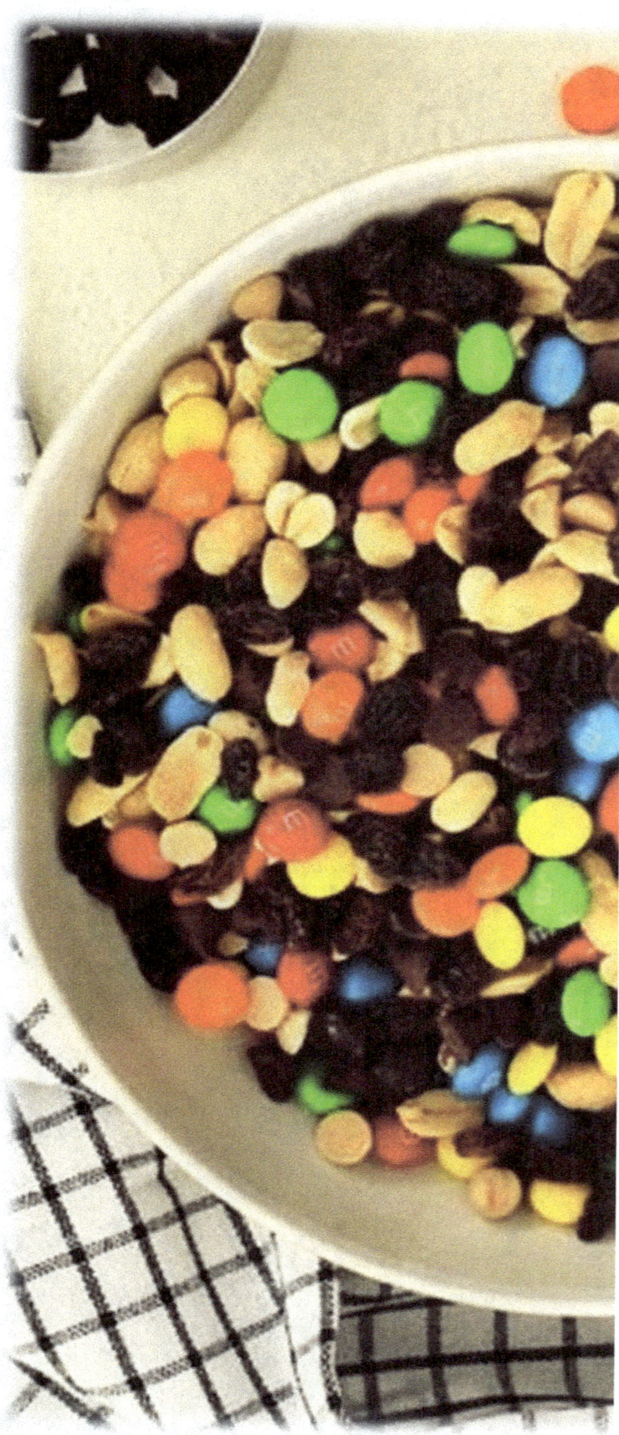

Dinner is often considered the main meal of the day, providing an opportunity to unwind and nourish the body after a busy day. In the context of the DASH (Dietary Approaches to Stop Hypertension) diet, dinner plays a crucial role in promoting heart health and overall well-being by incorporating nutrient-rich foods and balanced meals.

The dinner recipes featured in the DASH Diet Cookbook are designed to be delicious, satisfying, and easy to prepare, making them perfect for families and individuals alike. From flavorful main courses and hearty salads to comforting soups and vegetable-based dishes, these recipes offer a variety of options to suit different tastes and dietary preferences.

By incorporating DASH-friendly dinner recipes into your meal planning, you'll not only enjoy delicious and nutritious meals but also support your efforts to maintain a healthy lifestyle. Whether you're cooking for yourself, your family, or guests, the DASH Diet Cookbook has a range of dinner recipes to inspire your culinary creativity and nourish your body with wholesome ingredients.

Hummus and Veggie Sticks

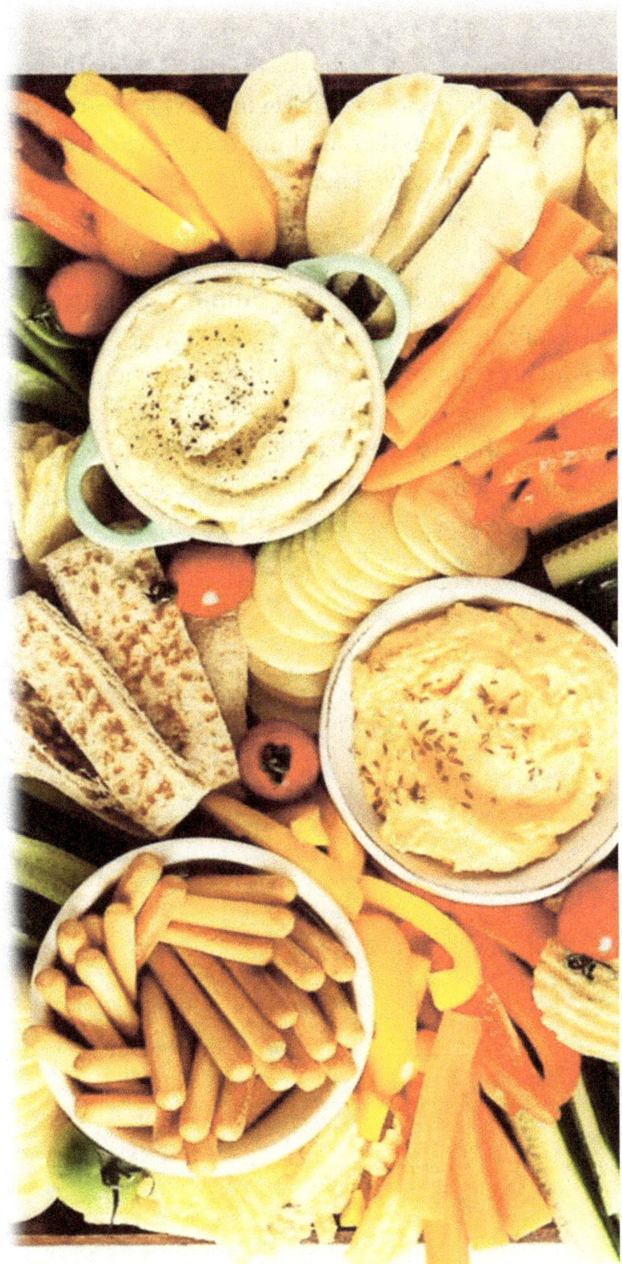

Ingredients:

- ❖ 1/2 cup homemade or store-bought hummus
- ❖ Assorted vegetable sticks (such as carrots, celery, bell peppers, cucumber, and cherry tomatoes)
- ❖ Optional: Whole grain crackers or pita bread, sliced

Procedures:

- ❖ Arrange the hummus in the center of a serving plate or bowl.
- ❖ Wash and prepare the assorted vegetable sticks by cutting them into manageable sizes.
- ❖ Arrange the vegetable sticks around the hummus, creating an attractive and colorful presentation.
- ❖ Serve immediately, along with whole grain crackers or pita bread slices if desired.

Nutritional Values (per serving):

- ❖ **Calories:** 150
- ❖ **Protein:** 5g
- ❖ **Carbohydrates:** 20g
- ❖ **Dietary Fiber:** 7g
- ❖ **Sugars:** 3g
- ❖ **Fat:** 7g
- ❖ **Saturated Fat:** 1g
- ❖ **Cholesterol:** 0mg
- ❖ **Sodium:** 300mg
- ❖ **Potassium:** 400mg
- ❖ **Calcium:** 50mg
- ❖ **Iron:** 2mg

- ❖ **Preparation Time:** 10 minutes
- ❖ **Cooking Time:** 0 minutes
- ❖ **Serving Unit:** 1 plate

Cooking Tips:

❖ Choose a variety of colorful vegetables to create an appealing and nutrient-rich snack.

❖ Opt for homemade hummus or choose a store-bought version with minimal added ingredients and low sodium content.

❖ Customize the hummus and vegetable sticks with additional toppings such as olives, feta cheese, or herbs for added flavor and nutrition.

❖ Keep the vegetable sticks refrigerated until ready to serve to maintain their crispness and freshness.

❖ For added convenience, pre-cut and wash the vegetables ahead of time and store them in an airtight container in the refrigerator until ready to serve.

Health Benefits:

❖ **Rich in Fiber:** Hummus and vegetable sticks are high in dietary fiber, which promotes digestive health, regulates blood sugar levels, and supports weight management by promoting feelings of fullness and reducing hunger cravings.

❖ **Nutrient-Dense:** Vegetables are rich in essential vitamins, minerals, and antioxidants, including vitamin C, vitamin A, potassium, and folate, which support immune function, vision health, and overall well-being.

❖ **Heart-Healthy Fats:** Hummus is made from chickpeas and olive oil, both of which are sources of heart-healthy monounsaturated fats, which help reduce inflammation and improve cholesterol levels.

❖ **Low in Calories:** Hummus and vegetable sticks are low in calories but high in volume, making them a satisfying and nutritious snack option that can support weight management goals.

❖ **Gluten-Free and Vegan-Friendly:** Hummus and vegetable sticks are naturally gluten-free and suitable for individuals following a vegan or plant-based diet, making them a versatile and inclusive snack option.

By incorporating this simple yet nutritious Hummus and Veggie Sticks snack into your meal rotation, you'll enjoy a delicious and satisfying way to boost your intake of vegetables and essential nutrients. Whether enjoyed as a midday snack, appetizer, or party platter, this recipe is sure to be a hit with friends and family alike.

Greek Yogurt with Berries

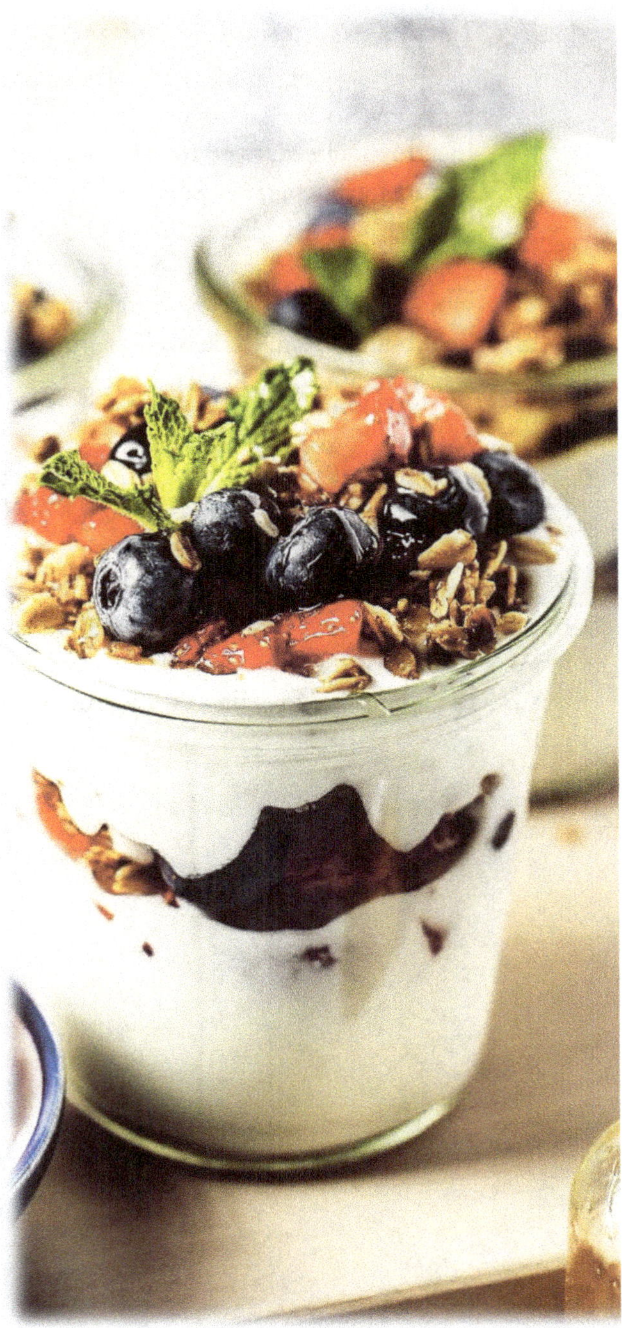

- ❖ **Preparation Time**: 5 minutes
- ❖ **Cooking Time**: 0 minutes
- ❖ **Serving Unit**: 1 bowl

Ingredients:

- ❖ 1/2 cup plain Greek yogurt
- ❖ ☐ 1/2 cup of mixed berries, including blackberries, raspberries, blueberries, and strawberries
- ❖ 1 tablespoon honey or maple syrup (optional)
- ❖ 1 tablespoon chopped nuts or granola (optional)
- ❖ Fresh mint leaves, for garnish (optional)

Procedures:

- ❖ Transfer the plain Greek yogurt into a dish for serving.
- ❖ Wash and prepare the mixed berries by rinsing them unqder cold water and patting them dry with a paper towel.
- ❖ Place the mixed berries in an arrangement on the Greek yogurt.
- ❖ Drizzle honey or maple syrup over the yogurt and berries, if desired, for added sweetness.
- ❖ Sprinkle chopped nuts or granola over the yogurt and berries for added texture and crunch, if desired.
- ❖ Garnish with fresh mint leaves for a burst of freshness and color, if desired.
- ❖ Serve immediately and enjoy!

Nutritional Values (per serving):

- ❖ **Calories**: 150
- ❖ **Protein**: 12g
- ❖ **Carbohydrates**: 20g
- ❖ **Dietary Fiber**: 4g
- ❖ **Sugars**: 14g
- ❖ **Fat**: 3g
- ❖ **Saturated Fat**: 1g
- ❖ **Cholesterol**: 10mg

- ❖ **Sodium**: 50mg
- ❖ **Potassium**: 250mg
- ❖ **Calcium**: 150mg
- ❖ **Iron**: 1mg

Cooking Tips:

- ❖ Use plain Greek yogurt with no added sugars or flavorings for a healthier option. Greek yogurt is thicker and creamier than regular yogurt, making it a delicious base for this dish.
- ❖ Customize the Greek yogurt with your favorite berries and toppings, such as sliced bananas, kiwi, or mango, for added flavor and variety.
- ❖ Choose fresh, ripe berries when available for the best flavor and texture. You can also use frozen berries if fresh ones are not in season.
- ❖ For added crunch and nutrition, sprinkle chopped nuts or granola over the yogurt and berries just before serving.
- ❖ Serve Greek yogurt with berries as a nutritious breakfast, snack, or dessert option that's quick and easy to prepare.

Health Benefits:

- ❖ **High in Protein:** Greek yogurt is a rich source of high-quality protein, which is essential for muscle repair and growth, as well as satiety, helping you feel full and satisfied.
- ❖ **Rich in Antioxidants:** Berries are packed with antioxidants, such as anthocyanins and flavonoids, which help fight inflammation, protect against oxidative stress, and reduce the risk of chronic diseases, including heart disease and cancer.
- ❖ **Probiotic-Rich:** Greek yogurt contains probiotics, beneficial bacteria that support gut health and digestion by promoting the growth of healthy bacteria in the gut.
- ❖ **Low in Added Sugars:** This dish is naturally sweetened with fruit and contains no added sugars, making it a healthier alternative to store-bought yogurt parfaits and desserts.
- ❖ **Calcium and Vitamin D:** Greek yogurt is a good source of calcium and vitamin D, which are essential for bone health and strength, as well as immune function and overall well-being.

By incorporating this simple yet nutritious Greek Yogurt with Berries dish into your meal rotation, you'll enjoy a delicious and satisfying way to boost your intake of protein, vitamins, minerals, and antioxidants. Whether enjoyed as a breakfast option, snack, or dessert, this recipe is sure to become a favorite in your culinary repertoire.

Homemade Trail Mix

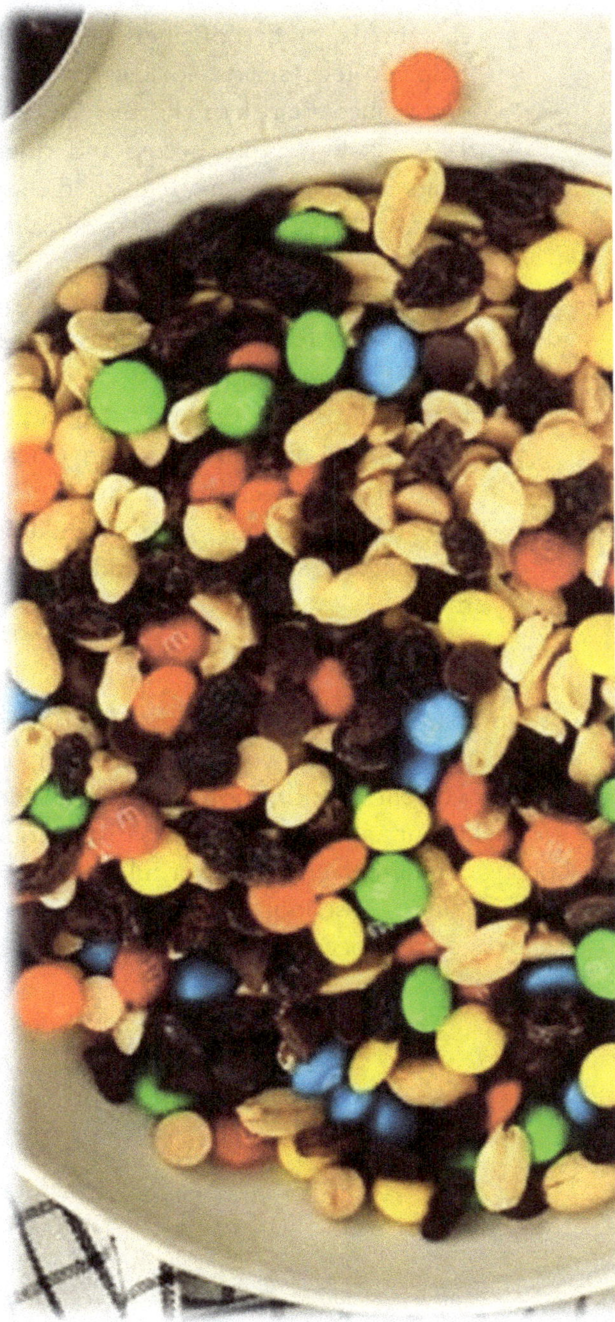

* **Preparation Time:** 5 minutes
* **Cooking Time:** 0 minutes
* **Serving Unit:** 1 cup

Ingredients:

* 1/2 cup raw almonds
* 1/2 cup raw cashews
* 1/2 cup raw walnuts
* 1/4 cup dried cranberries
* 1/4 cup raisins
* 1/4 cup chunks or chips of dark chocolate
* 1/4 cup pumpkin seeds (pepitas)
* Optional: Shredded coconut, banana chips, dried apricots, or any other favorite nuts, seeds, or dried fruits

Procedures:

* In a large mixing bowl, combine the raw almonds, cashews, walnuts, dried cranberries, raisins, dark chocolate chips or chunks, and pumpkin seeds.
* If desired, add any optional ingredients such as shredded coconut, banana chips, or dried apricots.
* Toss the ingredients together until they are evenly distributed throughout the trail mix.
* Transfer the homemade trail mix to an airtight container for storage.
* Serve the trail mix as a convenient and nutritious snack on-the-go.

Nutritional Values (per serving, approximately 1/4 cup):

* **Calories:** 200
* **Protein:** 6g
* **Carbohydrates:** 15g
* **Dietary Fiber:** 3g
* **Sugars:** 8g
* **Fat:** 14g
* **Saturated Fat:** 3g
* **Cholesterol:** 0mg

❖ **Sodium**: 5mg
❖ **Potassium**: 220mg
❖ **Calcium**: 40mg
❖ **Iron**: 1mg

Cooking Tips:

❖ Choose raw nuts and seeds for a healthier option, as they contain more nutrients and healthy fats compared to roasted and salted varieties.
❖ Customize the trail mix with your favorite nuts, seeds, and dried fruits for a personalized blend of flavors and textures.
❖ Keep portion sizes in mind when enjoying trail mix, as it can be calorie-dense. Aim to consume a serving size of approximately 1/4 cup at a time.
❖ Store homemade trail mix in an airtight container in a cool, dry place to maintain freshness and prevent spoilage.
❖ Consider portioning out individual servings of trail mix into small containers or resealable bags for convenient snacking on-the-go.

Health Benefits:

❖ **Nutrient-Rich:** Homemade trail mix is packed with essential nutrients, including protein, healthy fats, dietary fiber, vitamins, and minerals, which provide sustained energy and support overall health and well-being.
❖ **Heart-Healthy Fats:** Nuts and seeds in trail mix are rich in heart-healthy monounsaturated and polyunsaturated fats, which help reduce inflammation, improve cholesterol levels, and support cardiovascular health.
❖ **Antioxidant-Rich:** Dried fruits and dark chocolate in trail mix are rich in antioxidants, such as vitamins C and E, flavonoids, and polyphenols, which help protect against oxidative stress and reduce the risk of chronic diseases.
❖ **Fiber-Filled:** Nuts, seeds, and dried fruits in trail mix are high in dietary fiber, which promotes digestive health, regulates blood sugar levels, and supports weight management by promoting feelings of fullness and reducing hunger cravings.
❖ **Convenient and Portable:** Homemade trail mix is a convenient and portable snack option that can be enjoyed on-the-go, whether hiking, traveling, or simply as a midday pick-me-up.

By preparing this simple yet nutritious Homemade Trail Mix, you'll have a delicious and convenient snack option readily available to fuel your adventures and satisfy your cravings. Whether enjoyed as a hiking snack, office snack, or school snack, this versatile recipe is sure to become a staple in your snack repertoire.

Cucumber and Tomato Slices with Feta

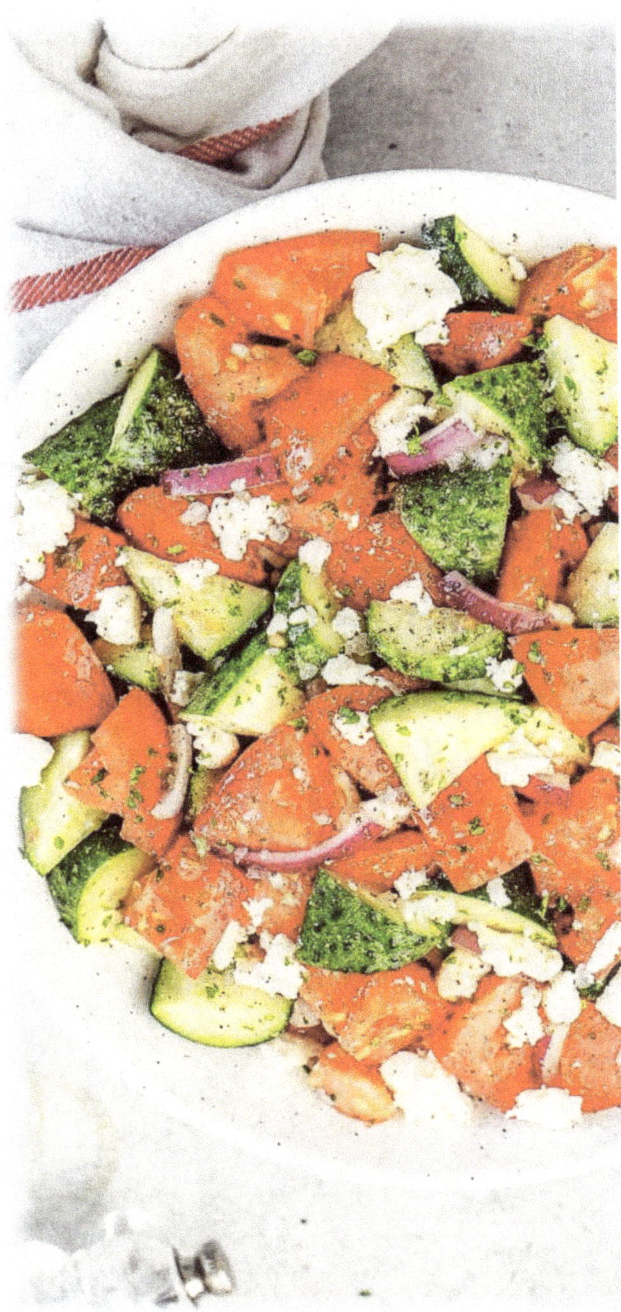

Ingredients:

- ❖ 1 large cucumber, thinly sliced
- ❖ 2 medium tomatoes, thinly sliced
- ❖ 1/4 cup crumbled feta cheese
- ❖ 2 tablespoons extra virgin olive oil
- ❖ 1 tablespoon balsamic vinegar or lemon juice
- ❖ 1 tablespoon chopped fresh basil or parsley
- ❖ Salt and pepper, to taste

Procedures:

- ❖ Arrange the thinly sliced cucumber and tomato slices on a serving plate, alternating them for an attractive presentation.
- ❖ Sprinkle crumbled feta cheese evenly over the cucumber and tomato slices.
- ❖ In a small bowl, whisk together the extra virgin olive oil and balsamic vinegar or lemon juice to make the dressing.
- ❖ Drizzle the dressing over the cucumber, tomato, and feta cheese.
- ❖ Sprinkle chopped fresh basil or parsley over the top of the salad.
- ❖ Season with salt and pepper to taste.
- ❖ Serve immediately and enjoy!

- ❖ **Preparation Time:** 10 minutes
- ❖ **Cooking Time:** 0 minutes
- ❖ **Serving Unit:** 1 plate

Nutritional Values (per serving):

- ❖ **Calories:** 150
- ❖ **Protein:** 5g
- ❖ **Carbohydrates:** 10g
- ❖ **Dietary Fiber:** 3g
- ❖ **Sugars:** 5g
- ❖ **Fat:** 10g
- ❖ **Saturated Fat:** 3g
- ❖ **Cholesterol:** 15mg

- ❖ **Sodium**: 300mg
- ❖ **Potassium**: 500mg
- ❖ **Calcium**: 150mg
- ❖ **Iron**: 1mg

Cooking Tips:

- ❖ Use ripe, firm tomatoes and crisp cucumbers for the best flavor and texture.
- ❖ Slice the cucumbers and tomatoes thinly and evenly for a consistent texture and easier eating.
- ❖ Customize the salad with additional ingredients such as red onion, olives, or avocado for added flavor and variety.
- ❖ For a creamier texture, mix the feta cheese with a small amount of Greek yogurt or sour cream before sprinkling it over the salad.
- ❖ Serve the cucumber and tomato slices with feta as a refreshing side dish or light lunch option.

Health Benefits:

- ❖ **Low in Calories:** Cucumber and tomato slices with feta are low in calories but high in volume, making them a satisfying and nutritious option for those watching their calorie intake.
- ❖ **Rich in Vitamins and Minerals:** Cucumbers and tomatoes are rich in essential vitamins and minerals, including vitamin C, vitamin K, potassium, and antioxidants, which support immune function, bone health, and overall well-being.
- ❖ **Heart-Healthy Fats:** Extra virgin olive oil used in the dressing provides heart-healthy monounsaturated fats, which help reduce inflammation and improve cholesterol levels.
- ❖ **Protein-Rich:** Feta cheese adds a boost of protein to the salad, which is essential for muscle repair and growth, as well as satiety, helping you feel full and satisfied.
- ❖ **Hydrating:** Cucumbers are high in water content, which helps keep you hydrated and promotes healthy skin and digestion.

By preparing this simple yet flavorful Cucumber and Tomato Slices with Feta salad, you'll enjoy a delicious and nutritious dish that's perfect for any occasion. Whether served as a side dish at a barbecue, picnic, or potluck, or enjoyed as a light lunch or snack at home, this versatile recipe is sure to become a favorite in your culinary repertoire.

4

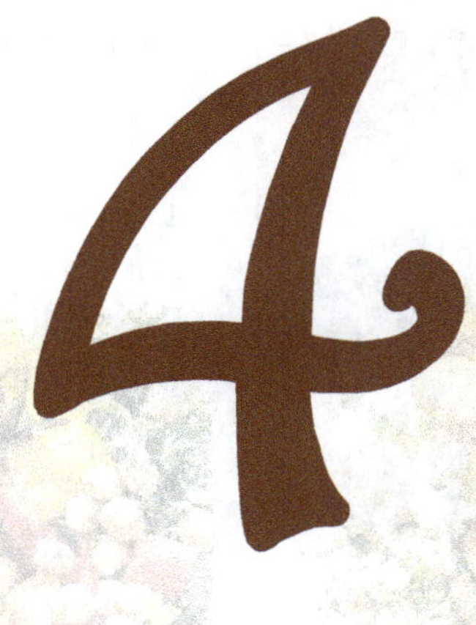

Introduction to Soup and Salad Recipes

Introduction to Soup and Salad Recipes

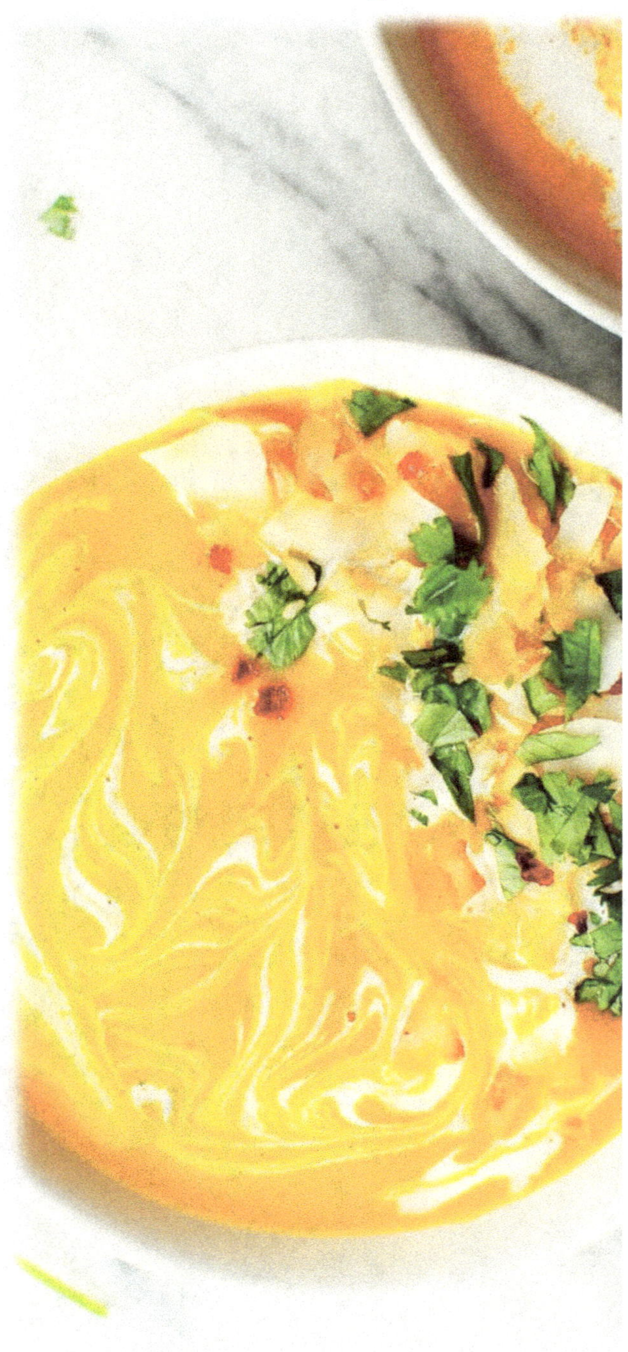

Soup and salad are versatile dishes that can be enjoyed as appetizers, light meals, or even hearty main courses. In the context of the DASH (Dietary Approaches to Stop Hypertension) diet, soups and salads offer an excellent opportunity to incorporate nutrient-rich ingredients such as vegetables, lean proteins, whole grains, and legumes, which are essential for supporting heart health and overall well-being.

The soup and salad recipes featured in the DASH Diet Cookbook are designed to be flavorful, satisfying, and packed with wholesome ingredients that nourish the body and promote good health. From comforting soups and vibrant salads to refreshing gazpachos and hearty chilis, these recipes offer a wide range of options to suit different tastes and dietary preferences.

By incorporating DASH-friendly soup and salad recipes into your meal planning, you'll not only enjoy delicious and nutritious meals but also support your efforts to maintain a balanced and heart-healthy diet. Whether you're looking for a light lunch, a comforting dinner, or a flavorful side dish, the DASH Diet Cookbook has you covered with a variety of soup and salad recipes to suit every occasion.

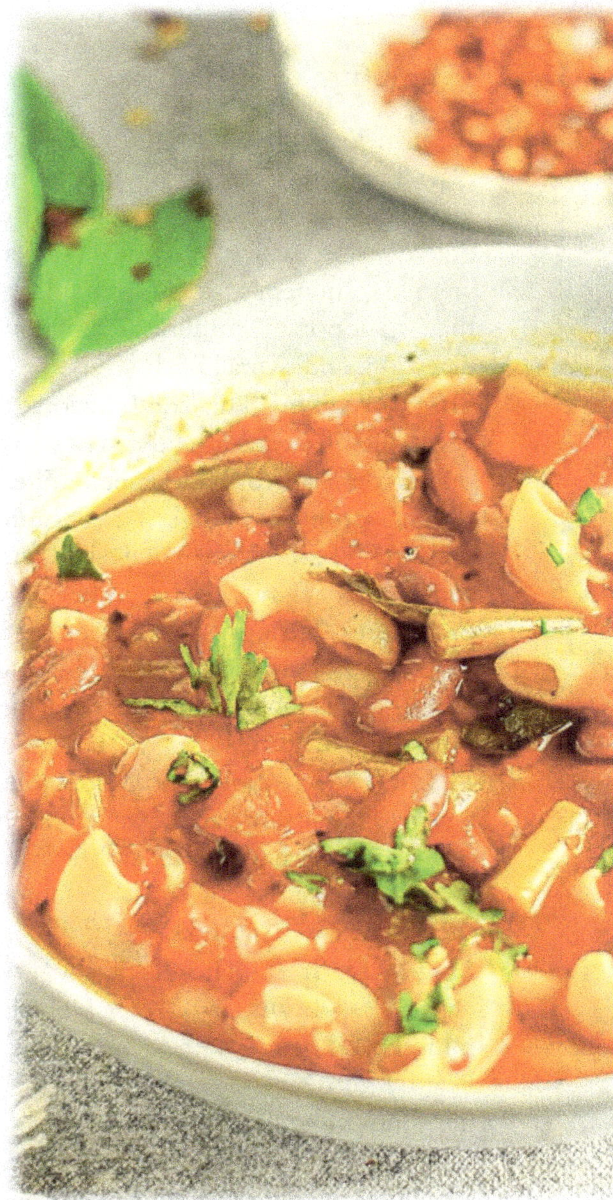

- ❖ **Preparation Time:** 15 minutes
- ❖ **Cooking Time:** 30 minutes
- ❖ **Serving Unit:** 1 bowl

Ingredients:

- ❖ 1 tablespoon olive oil
- ❖ 1 onion, diced
- ❖ 2 cloves garlic, minced
- ❖ 2 carrots, diced
- ❖ 2 celery stalks, diced
- ❖ 1 zucchini, diced
- ❖ 1 cup of green beans, chopped into small pieces after trimming
- ❖ 1 can (15 ounces) diced tomatoes
- ❖ 6 cups vegetable broth
- ❖ 1 can (15 ounces) cannellini beans, drained and rinsed
- ❖ A cup of little pasta, such elbow macaroni or tiny shells
- ❖ 1 teaspoon dried oregano
- ❖ 1 teaspoon dried basil
- ❖ Salt and pepper, to taste
- ❖ Grated Parmesan cheese, for serving (optional)
- ❖ Fresh basil leaves, for garnish (optional)

Procedures:

- ❖ Heat the olive oil in a big saucepan or Dutch oven over medium heat.
- ❖ Add the diced onion and minced garlic to the pot and sauté for 2-3 minutes, or until softened and fragrant.
- ❖ Add the diced carrots, celery, zucchini, and green beans to the pot, and cook for an additional 5 minutes, stirring occasionally.
- ❖ Pour in the diced tomatoes and vegetable broth, and bring the soup to a simmer.
- ❖ Add the drained and rinsed cannellini beans, small pasta, dried oregano, and dried basil to the pot, and stir to combine.
- ❖ Add salt and pepper to taste when preparing the soup.
- ❖ Allow the soup to simmer for 15-20 minutes, or until the vegetables are tender and the pasta is cooked al dente.

- ❖ Taste and adjust seasoning as needed.
- ❖ Transfer the minestrone soup into dishes for dishing.
- ❖ If preferred, garnish with freshly chopped basil leaves and grated Parmesan cheese.
- ❖ Serve hot and enjoy!

Nutritional Values (per serving):

- ❖ **Calories**: 250
- ❖ **Protein**: 10g
- ❖ **Carbohydrates**: 40g
- ❖ **Dietary Fiber**: 8g
- ❖ **Sugars**: 8g
- ❖ **Fat**: 5g
- ❖ **Saturated Fat**: 1g
- ❖ **Cholesterol**: 0mg
- ❖ **Sodium**: 800mg
- ❖ **Potassium**: 600mg
- ❖ **Calcium**: 100mg
- ❖ **Iron**: 3mg

Cooking Tips:

- ❖ Customize the soup by adding additional vegetables such as diced potatoes, cabbage, spinach, or kale for added flavor and nutrition.
- ❖ Use low-sodium vegetable broth to control the sodium content of the soup, especially if you are watching your salt intake.
- ❖ For a protein boost, add cooked chicken, turkey, or tofu to the soup along with the vegetables.
- ❖ Cook the pasta separately and add it to the soup just before serving to prevent it from becoming too soft and mushy.
- ❖ Store leftover minestrone soup in an airtight container in the refrigerator for up to 3-4 days, or freeze it for longer storage.

Health Benefits:

- ❖ **Rich in Vegetables:** Minestrone soup is packed with a variety of vegetables, including carrots, celery, zucchini, and green beans, which provide essential vitamins, minerals, and antioxidants that support immune function, digestion, and overall health.
- ❖ **High in Fiber:** The combination of vegetables, beans, and pasta in minestrone soup provides dietary fiber, which promotes digestive health, regulates blood sugar levels, and supports weight management by promoting feelings of fullness and reducing hunger cravings. decreasing hunger cravings and encouraging sensations of fullness.
- ❖ **Low in Calories and Fat:** Minestrone soup is a low-calorie and low-fat option that's rich in flavor and satisfaction, making it suitable for those watching their calorie and fat intake.
- ❖ **Heart-Healthy**: The inclusion of vegetables, beans, and olive oil in minestrone soup provides heart-healthy nutrients such as antioxidants, monounsaturated fats, and soluble fiber, which help reduce inflammation, lower cholesterol levels, and improve cardiovascular health.
- ❖ **Versatile and Nutritious:** Minestrone soup can be customized with a variety of ingredients to suit different tastes and dietary preferences, making it a versatile and nutritious option for individuals and families alike.

Kale Caesar Salad with Grilled Chicken

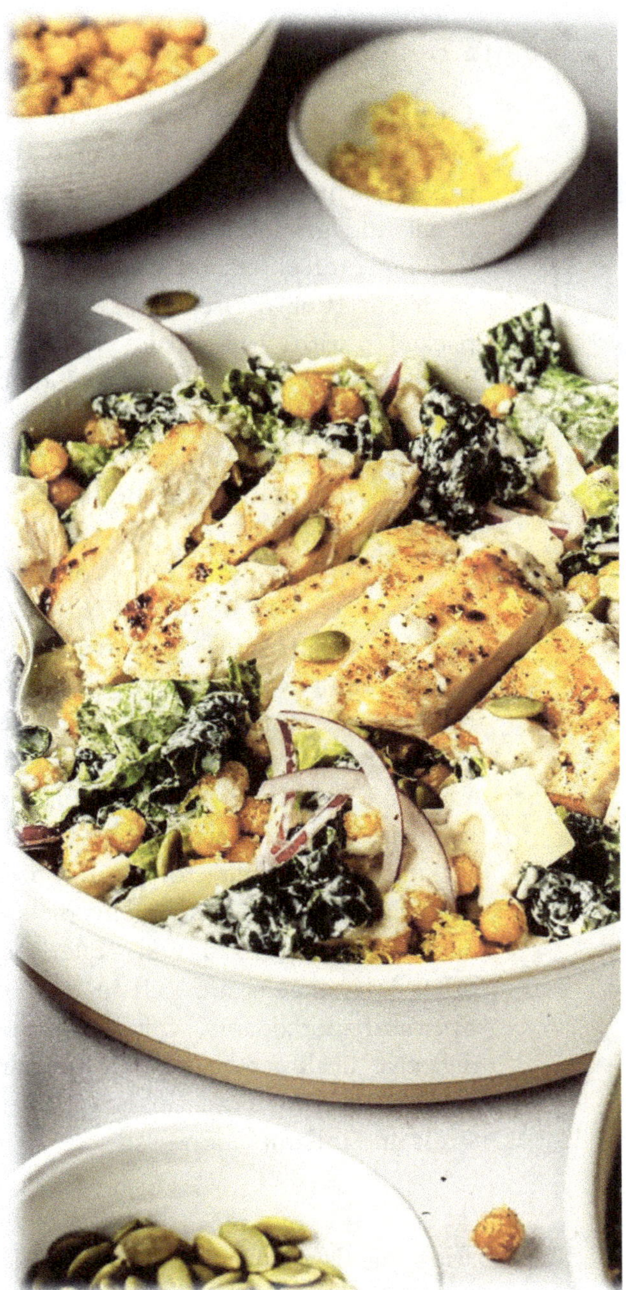

- ❖ **Preparation Time:** 20 minutes
- ❖ **Cooking Time:** 15 minutes
- ❖ **Serving Unit:** 1 plate

Ingredients:

- ❖ 2 cups of finely chopped, stem-free kale leaves
- ❖ 1 grilled chicken breast, sliced
- ❖ 1/4 cup Caesar salad dressing
- ❖ 1/4 cup grated Parmesan cheese
- ❖ 1/4 cup croutons
- ❖ Lemon wedges, for garnish (optional)

For the Grilled Chicken:

- ❖ 1 boneless, skinless chicken breast
- ❖ 1 tablespoon olive oil
- ❖ 1 teaspoon garlic powder
- ❖ 1 teaspoon dried oregano
- ❖ Salt and pepper, to taste

Procedures; For the Grilled Chicken:

- ❖ Preheat grill to medium-high heat.
- ❖ In a small bowl, mix together olive oil, garlic powder, dried oregano, salt, and pepper.
- ❖ Rub the seasoning mixture over the chicken breast.
- ❖ Grill the chicken breast for 6-7 minutes on each side, or until cooked through and no longer pink in the center.
- ❖ Remove the chicken from the grill and let it rest for a few minutes before slicing.

For the Salad:

- ❖ In a large mixing bowl, add chopped kale leaves.
- ❖ Drizzle Caesar salad dressing over the kale leaves and toss to coat evenly.
- ❖ Add sliced grilled chicken breast to the bowl.

❖ Top the salad with croutons and grated Parmesan cheese.
❖ Toss the salad gently to combine all the ingredients.
❖ Spoon the salad onto a platter.
❖ Garnish with lemon wedges, if desired.
❖ Serve immediately and enjoy!

Nutritional Values (per serving):

❖ **Calories**: 350
❖ **Protein**: 30g
❖ **Carbohydrates**: 10g
❖ **Dietary Fiber**: 2g
❖ **Sugars**: 2g
❖ **Fat**: 20g
❖ **Saturated Fat**: 5g
❖ **Cholesterol**: 80mg
❖ **Sodium**: 600mg
❖ **Potassium**: 500mg
❖ **Calcium**: 200mg
❖ **Iron**: 2mg

Cooking Tips:

❖ Massage the kale leaves with a little olive oil before adding the dressing to help tenderize them and reduce bitterness.
❖ For added flavor, sprinkle some freshly squeezed lemon juice over the salad just before serving.
❖ Use homemade or store-bought Caesar salad dressing according to your preference. Look for a dressing with natural ingredients and minimal added sugars and preservatives.
❖ Customize the salad by adding additional toppings such as cherry tomatoes, avocado slices, or bacon bits for extra flavor and texture.
❖ Use leftover grilled chicken or store-bought rotisserie chicken to save time and simplify meal preparation.

Health Benefits:

❖ **High in Protein**: Grilled chicken breast provides a lean source of protein, which is essential for muscle repair and growth, as well as satiety, helping you feel full and satisfied.
❖ **Nutrient-Rich Greens**: Kale is packed with essential vitamins, minerals, and antioxidants, including vitamin A, vitamin C, vitamin K, calcium, and potassium, which support immune function, bone health, and overall well-being.
❖ **Heart-Healthy Fats**: Olive oil and Parmesan cheese in the Caesar salad dressing provide heart-healthy monounsaturated fats, which help reduce inflammation and improve cholesterol levels.
❖ **Low in Carbohydrates**: This salad is low in carbohydrates and sugars, making it suitable for individuals following low-carb or ketogenic diets.
❖ **Fiber and Antioxidants**: Kale and other leafy greens are rich in dietary fiber and antioxidants, which promote digestive health, regulate blood sugar levels, and protect against oxidative stress and inflammation.

By preparing this flavorful and nutritious Kale Caesar Salad with Grilled Chicken, you'll enjoy a delicious and satisfying meal that's packed with wholesome ingredients and flavor. Whether enjoyed as a light lunch, a hearty dinner, or a post-workout meal, this salad is sure to become a favorite in your meal rotation.

Butternut Squash Soup

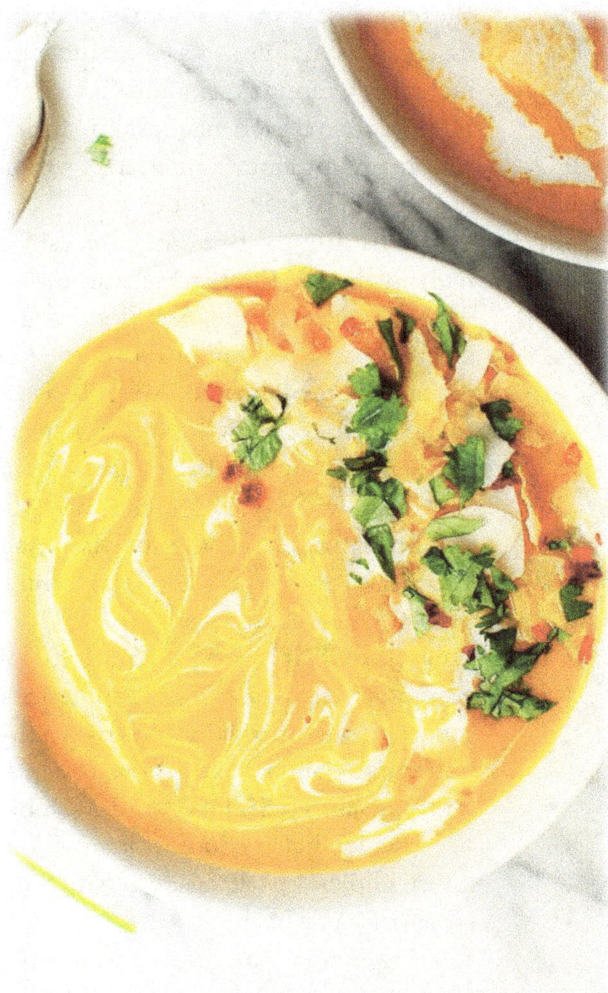

- ❖ **Preparation Time**: 15 minutes
- ❖ **Cooking Time**: 45 minutes
- ❖ **Serving Unit**: 1 bowl

Ingredients:

- ❖ 1 medium butternut squash, peeled, seeded, and diced
- ❖ 1 onion, diced
- ❖ 2 cloves garlic, minced
- ❖ 2 carrots, diced
- ❖ 2 celery stalks, diced
- ❖ 4 cups vegetable broth
- ❖ 1 teaspoon dried thyme
- ❖ 1/2 teaspoon ground cinnamon
- ❖ 1/4 teaspoon ground nutmeg
- ❖ Salt and pepper, to taste
- ❖ 2 tablespoons olive oil
- ❖ Optional garnishes: Fresh parsley, pumpkin seeds, Greek yogurt, or sour cream

Procedures:

- ❖ In a big saucepan, warm up the olive oil over medium heat.
- ❖ Add the minced garlic and chopped onion to the saucepan and sauté for two to three minutes, or until aromatic and softened.
- ❖ Add diced carrots and celery to the pot, and cook for an additional 5 minutes, stirring occasionally.
- ❖ Add diced butternut squash to the pot, along with dried thyme, ground cinnamon, and ground nutmeg. Stir to combine.
- ❖ Pour vegetable broth into the pot and bring the soup to a simmer.
- ❖ Reduce heat to low, cover, and let the soup simmer for 30-35 minutes, or until the butternut squash is tender.
- ❖ Once the squash is cooked through, use an immersion blender to puree the soup until smooth and creamy. On the other hand, put the soup to a blender and process until smooth, working in batches.
- ❖ Season the soup with salt and pepper to taste Add salt and pepper to taste when preparing the soup.
- ❖ Transfer the butternut squash soup into dishes for dishing.

❖ Garnish with fresh parsley, pumpkin seeds, Greek yogurt, or sour cream, if desired.
❖ Serve hot and enjoy!

Nutritional Values (per serving):

❖ **Calories**: 150
❖ **Protein**: 3g
❖ **Carbohydrates**: 25g
❖ **Dietary Fiber**: 5g
❖ **Sugars**: 6g
❖ **Fat**: 5g
❖ **Saturated Fat**: 1g
❖ **Cholesterol**: 0mg
❖ **Sodium**: 600mg
❖ **Potassium**: 700mg
❖ **Calcium**: 100mg
❖ **Iron**: 2mg

Cooking Tips:

❖ Choose a medium-sized butternut squash that feels heavy for its size and has a firm, unblemished skin.
❖ To make peeling easier, slice off both ends of the squash, then use a vegetable peeler to remove the skin in downward strokes.
❖ For added flavor, roast the diced butternut squash in the oven at 400°F (200°C) for 20-25 minutes before adding it to the soup.
❖ Customize the soup with additional spices such as ginger, cumin, or curry powder for a more complex flavor profile.
❖ Use low-sodium vegetable broth to control the sodium content of the soup, especially if you are watching your salt intake.

Health Benefits:

❖ **Rich in Vitamins and Minerals:** Butternut squash is a rich source of essential vitamins and minerals, including vitamin A, vitamin C, vitamin E, potassium, and magnesium, which support immune function, vision health, and overall well-being.
❖ **High in Fiber:** Butternut squash is high in dietary fiber, which promotes digestive health, regulates blood sugar levels, and supports weight management by promoting feelings of fullness and reducing hunger cravings.
❖ **Low in Calories:** Butternut squash soup is low in calories but high in volume, making it a satisfying and nutritious option for those watching their calorie intake.
❖ **Heart-Healthy:** The inclusion of vegetables and olive oil in butternut squash soup provides heart-healthy nutrients such as antioxidants, monounsaturated fats, and soluble fiber, which help reduce inflammation, lower cholesterol levels, and improve cardiovascular health.
❖ **Versatile and Nutritious:** Butternut squash soup can be customized with a variety of ingredients and spices to suit different tastes and dietary preferences, making it a versatile and nutritious option for individuals and families alike.

By preparing this flavorful and comforting Butternut Squash Soup, you'll enjoy a delicious and nutritious dish that's perfect for warming up on chilly days. Whether enjoyed as a light lunch, a satisfying dinner, or a starter for a special meal, this soup is sure to become a favorite in your culinary repertoire.

Caprese Salad with Balsamic Glaze

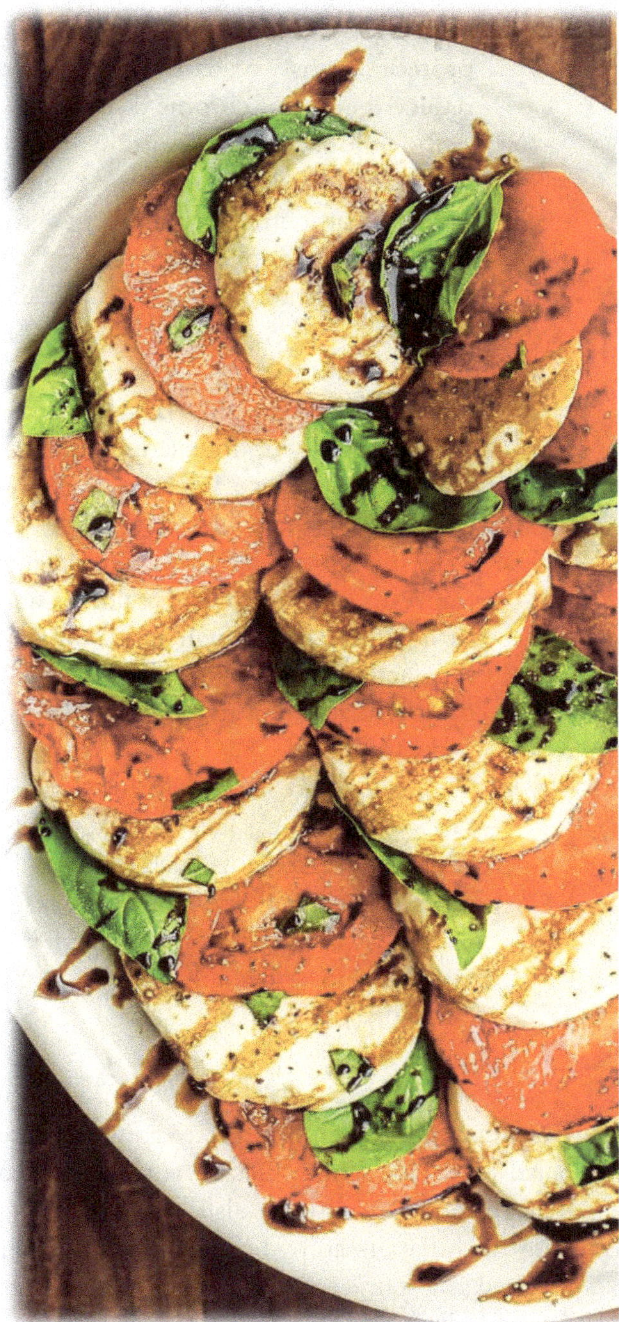

- ❖ **Preparation Time:** 10 minutes
- ❖ **Cooking Time:** 5 minutes
- ❖ **Serving Unit:** 1 plate

Ingredients:

- ❖ 1 large ripe tomato, sliced
- ❖ 1 ball fresh mozzarella cheese, sliced
- ❖ Fresh basil leaves
- ❖ Balsamic glaze
- ❖ Extra virgin olive oil
- ❖ Salt and pepper, to taste

For the Balsamic Glaze:

- ❖ 1/2 cup balsamic vinegar
- ❖ 2 tablespoons honey or maple syrup (optional)

Procedures; For the Balsamic Glaze:

- ❖ Simmer the balsamic vinegar in a small saucepan over medium heat.
- ❖ If using honey or maple syrup, add it to the vinegar and stir until dissolved.
- ❖ Reduce heat to low and let the vinegar simmer gently for 5-7 minutes, or until it has thickened and reduced by half.
- ❖ Remove the saucepan from heat and let the balsamic glaze cool to room temperature. As it cools, it will get thicker yet.

For the Salad:

- ❖ Arrange sliced tomatoes and mozzarella cheese alternately on a serving plate.
- ❖ Place a few fresh basil leaves in between the mozzarella and tomato slices.
- ❖ Drizzle balsamic glaze and extra virgin olive oil over the salad.
- ❖ Season with salt and pepper to taste.

❖ Serve immediately and enjoy!

Nutritional Values (per serving):

- **Calories**: 200
- **Protein**: 10g
- **Carbohydrates**: 15g
- **Dietary Fiber**: 2g
- **Sugars**: 10g
- **Fat**: 10g
- **Saturated Fat**: 5g
- **Cholesterol**: 25mg
- **Sodium**: 300mg
- **Potassium**: 400mg
- **Calcium**: 200mg
- **Iron**: 1mg

Cooking Tips:

- Choose ripe, flavorful tomatoes and fresh mozzarella cheese for the best taste and texture.
- If fresh basil is not available, you can use dried basil or substitute with fresh spinach leaves or arugula for added flavor and nutrition.
- Make sure the balsamic glaze has cooled to room temperature before drizzling it over the salad to prevent wilting the fresh basil leaves.
- To enhance the flavor of the salad, you can sprinkle some freshly ground black pepper or a pinch of Italian seasoning over the tomatoes and mozzarella cheese.
- Serve the Caprese salad as a refreshing appetizer, side dish, or light lunch option, paired with crusty bread or a bowl of soup.

Health Benefits:

- **Rich in Antioxidants**: Tomatoes and fresh basil in Caprese salad are rich in antioxidants, including vitamin C, vitamin A, and flavonoids, which help protect against oxidative stress and reduce the risk of chronic diseases.
- **Good Source of Protein**: Fresh mozzarella cheese provides a good source of protein, which is essential for muscle repair and growth, as well as satiety, helping you feel full and satisfied.
- **Heart-Healthy Fats**: Extra virgin olive oil used in the salad provides heart-healthy monounsaturated fats, which help reduce inflammation and improve cholesterol levels.
- **Low in Calories and Carbohydrates**: Caprese salad is low in calories and carbohydrates but high in flavor and satisfaction, making it a nutritious option for those watching their calorie and carb intake.
- **Versatile and Refreshing**: Caprese salad can be customized with additional ingredients such as avocado slices, olives, or roasted red peppers for added flavor and variety, making it a versatile and refreshing option for any occasion.

By preparing this simple yet elegant Caprese Salad with Balsamic Glaze, you'll enjoy a delicious and nutritious dish that's bursting with fresh flavors and vibrant colors. Whether enjoyed as a starter, side dish, or light meal, this classic Italian salad is sure to become a favorite in your culinary repertoire.

5

Introduction to Side Dish Recipes

Introduction to Side Dish Recipes

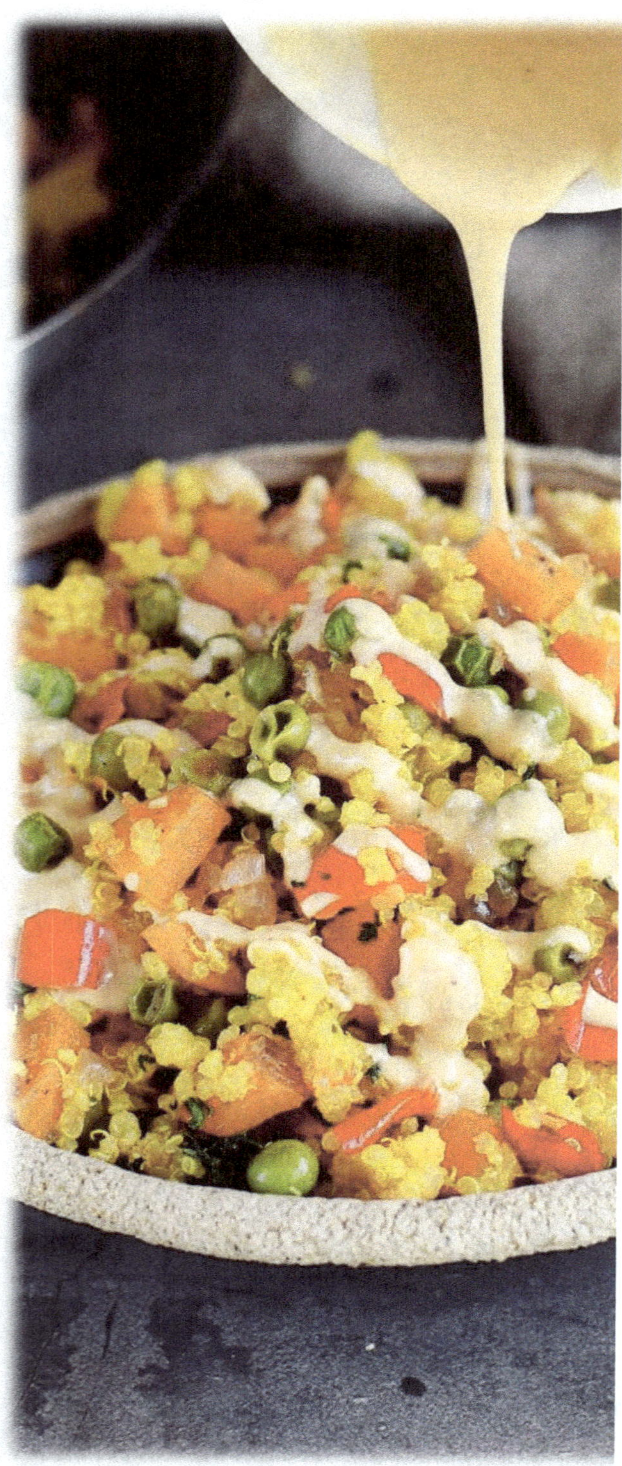

Side dishes are the unsung heroes of any meal, adding depth, flavor, and variety to the dining experience. In the context of the DASH (Dietary Approaches to Stop Hypertension) diet, side dishes play a crucial role in helping individuals meet their nutritional needs while adhering to heart-healthy guidelines. From vibrant vegetable medleys and wholesome grain salads to flavorful bean dishes and satisfying potato recipes, side dishes offer endless possibilities for incorporating nutrient-rich ingredients into the diet.

The side dish recipes featured in the DASH Diet Cookbook are designed to complement main courses while providing a balanced and nutritious accompaniment. Whether you're looking for a simple side salad, a hearty grain dish, or a flavorful vegetable medley, you'll find a variety of options to suit your taste preferences and dietary requirements.

By incorporating DASH-friendly side dish recipes into your meal planning, you'll not only enhance the flavor and appeal of your meals but also support your efforts to maintain a healthy and balanced diet. Whether served alongside a lean protein, a whole grain, or a plant-based entrée, these side dishes are sure to elevate your dining experience and contribute to your overall health and well-being.

Garlic Roasted Brussels Sprouts

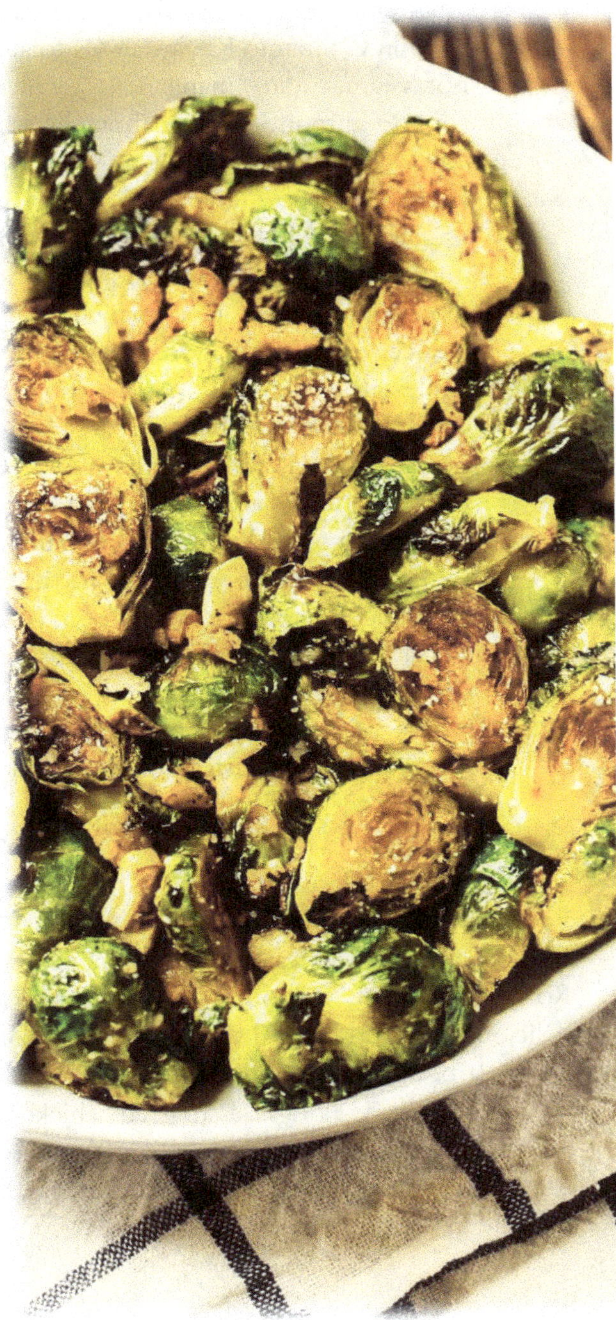

Ingredients:

- ❖ 1 pound of halved and trimmed Brussels sprouts
- ❖ 3 tablespoons olive oil
- ❖ 4 cloves garlic, minced
- ❖ Salt and pepper, to taste
- ❖ Optional: Grated Parmesan cheese, lemon zest, or balsamic glaze for serving

Procedures:

- ❖ Adjust the oven temperature to 400°F (200°C) and place parchment paper on a baking pan.
- ❖ Brussels sprouts cut in half should be uniformly covered after being tossed in a big mixing basin with chopped garlic and olive oil.
- ❖ Season the Brussels sprouts with salt and pepper to taste, and toss again to combine.
- ❖ Arrange the Brussels sprouts on the baking sheet that has been preheated in a single layer.
- ❖ Roast the Brussels sprouts in the preheated oven for 20 to 25 minutes, tossing them halfway through, or until they are soft and caramelized.
- ❖ Once roasted, remove the Brussels sprouts from the oven and transfer them to a serving plate.
- ❖ Optional: Sprinkle grated Parmesan cheese, lemon zest, or drizzle balsamic glaze over the roasted Brussels sprouts before serving.
- ❖ Serve hot and enjoy!

- ❖ **Preparation Time:** 10 minutes
- ❖ **Cooking Time:** 25 minutes
- ❖ **Serving Unit:** 1 plate

Nutritional Values (per serving):

- ❖ **Calories**: 150
- ❖ **Protein**: 5g
- ❖ **Carbohydrates**: 10g
- ❖ **Dietary Fiber**: 5g
- ❖ **Sugars**: 2g
- ❖ **Fat**: 10g
- ❖ **Saturated Fat**: 1g
- ❖ **Cholesterol**: 0mg
- ❖ **Sodium**: 30mg
- ❖ **Potassium**: 500mg
- ❖ **Calcium**: 50mg
- ❖ **Iron**: 2mg

Cooking Tips:

- ❖ Choose firm and fresh Brussels sprouts for the best flavor and texture.
- ❖ Make sure to trim the stem end of the Brussels sprouts and remove any discolored outer leaves before halving them.
- ❖ To ensure even roasting, spread the Brussels sprouts in a single layer on the baking sheet without overcrowding.
- ❖ For extra flavor, add a sprinkle of red pepper flakes or smoked paprika to the Brussels sprouts before roasting.
- ❖ For added richness, toss the roasted Brussels sprouts with crispy cooked bacon or pancetta before serving.

Health Benefits:

- ❖ High in Fiber: Brussels sprouts are a good source of dietary fiber, which promotes digestive health, regulates blood sugar levels, and supports weight management by promoting feelings of fullness and reducing hunger cravings.
- ❖ Rich in Vitamins and Minerals: Brussels sprouts are rich in essential vitamins and minerals, including vitamin C, vitamin K, vitamin A, folate, potassium, and manganese, which support immune function, bone health, and overall well-being.
- ❖ Heart-Healthy: Garlic and olive oil used in the recipe provide heart-healthy nutrients such as antioxidants and monounsaturated fats, which help reduce inflammation, improve cholesterol levels, and support cardiovascular health.
- ❖ Low in Calories: Garlic roasted Brussels sprouts are low in calories but high in flavor and satisfaction, making them a nutritious option for those watching their calorie intake.
- ❖ Versatile and Nutritious: Brussels sprouts can be customized with a variety of seasonings and toppings to suit different tastes and dietary preferences, making them a versatile and nutritious side dish for any meal.

By preparing this simple yet flavorful Garlic Roasted Brussels Sprouts, you'll enjoy a delicious and nutritious dish that's perfect for adding a pop of color and flavor to any meal. Whether served alongside roasted chicken, grilled fish, or as a standalone side dish, these roasted Brussels sprouts are sure to become a favorite in your meal rotation.

Quinoa Pilaf with Mixed Vegetables

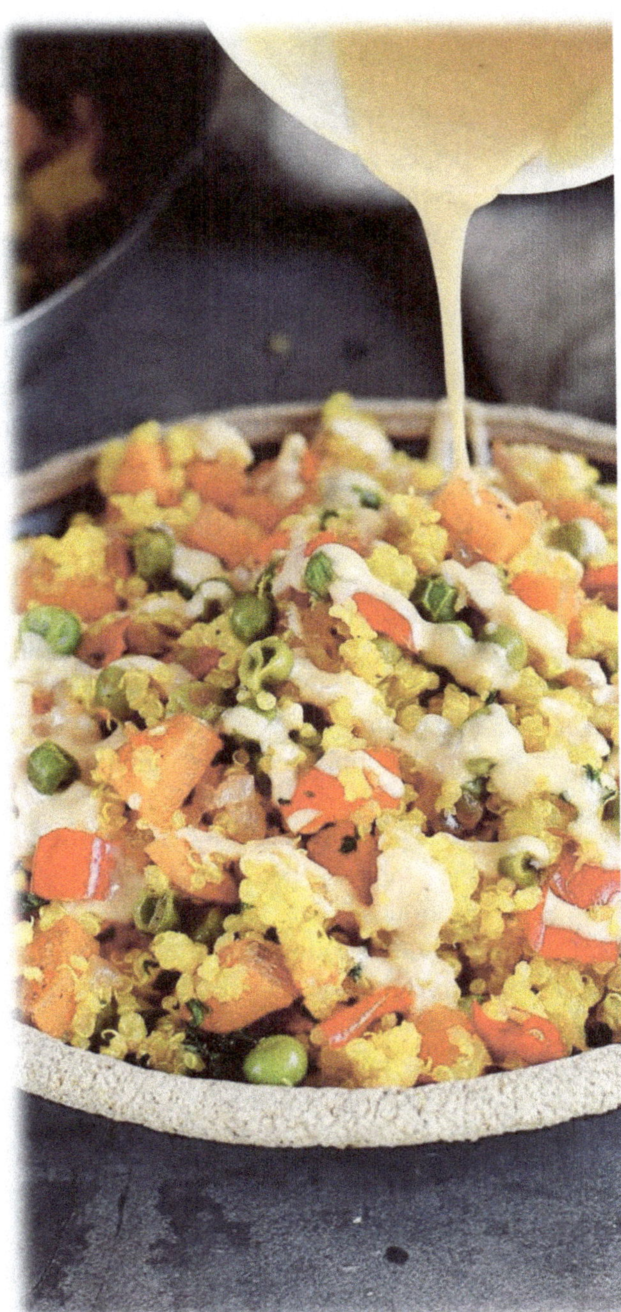

Ingredients:

- 1 cup quinoa, rinsed
- 2 cups vegetable broth or water
- 1 tablespoon olive oil
- 1 small onion, diced
- 2 cloves garlic, minced
- 1 carrot, diced
- 1 bell pepper, diced (any color)
- 1 zucchini, diced
- 1 cup frozen peas
- 1 teaspoon dried thyme
- Salt and pepper, to taste
- Optional: Fresh herbs (such as parsley or cilantro) for garnish

Procedures:

- Elevate the vegetable broth or water to a boil in a medium-sized saucepan.
- Add the rinsed quinoa to the saucepan, reduce heat to low, cover, and simmer for 15-20 minutes, or until the quinoa is cooked and the liquid is absorbed. After removing from the heat and covering for five minutes, fluff with a fork.
- Heat the olive oil in a big pan over medium heat while the quinoa cooks.
- Add diced onion and minced garlic to the skillet and sauté for 2-3 minutes, or until softened and fragrant.
- Add diced carrot, bell pepper, and zucchini to the skillet, and cook for an additional 5 minutes, stirring occasionally.
- Stir in the frozen peas and dried thyme, and cook for another 2-3 minutes, or until the vegetables are tender.

- **Preparation Time:** 15 minutes
- **Cooking Time:** 20 minutes
- **Serving Unit:** 1 plate

- ❖ Once the quinoa is cooked, add it to the skillet with the cooked vegetables, and toss to combine.
- ❖ Season the quinoa pilaf with salt and pepper to taste.
- ❖ Transfer the quinoa pilaf to a serving plate or bowl.
- ❖ Garnish with fresh herbs, if desired.
- ❖ Serve hot and enjoy!

Nutritional Values (per serving):

- ❖ Calories: 250
- ❖ Protein: 8g
- ❖ Carbohydrates: 40g
- ❖ Dietary Fiber: 8g
- ❖ Sugars: 5g
- ❖ Fat: 7g
- ❖ Saturated Fat: 1g
- ❖ Cholesterol: 0mg
- ❖ Sodium: 600mg
- ❖ Potassium: 600mg
- ❖ Calcium: 50mg
- ❖ Iron: 3mg

Cooking Tips:

- ❖ Rinse quinoa under cold water before cooking to remove any bitterness or residue.
- ❖ Use a vegetable broth instead of water to cook the quinoa for added flavor.
- ❖ Feel free to customize the vegetables based on what you have on hand or your personal preferences. Other options include broccoli, cauliflower, mushrooms, or spinach.
- ❖ Add a squeeze of fresh lemon juice or a drizzle of balsamic glaze over the quinoa pilaf for extra flavor.

- ❖ For a protein boost, add cooked chickpeas, tofu, or grilled chicken to the quinoa pilaf before serving.

Health Benefits:

- ❖ **High in Protein**: Quinoa is a complete protein, meaning it contains all nine essential amino acids, making it an excellent plant-based protein source for vegetarians and vegans.
- ❖ **Rich in Fiber**: Quinoa and mixed vegetables in this pilaf are high in dietary fiber, which promotes digestive health, regulates blood sugar levels, and supports weight management by promoting feelings of fullness and reducing hunger cravings.
- ❖ **Nutrient-Rich**: Quinoa and mixed vegetables are rich in essential vitamins, minerals, and antioxidants, including vitamin A, vitamin C, vitamin K, potassium, magnesium, and folate, which support immune function, bone health, and overall well-being.
- ❖ **Heart-Healthy Fats**: Olive oil used in the recipe provides heart-healthy monounsaturated fats, which help reduce inflammation and improve cholesterol levels.
- ❖ **Low in Calories**: Quinoa pilaf with mixed vegetables is low in calories but high in nutrients and flavor, making it a satisfying and nutritious option for those watching their calorie intake.

By preparing this flavorful and nutritious Quinoa Pilaf with Mixed Vegetables, you'll enjoy a delicious and satisfying dish that's perfect for lunch, dinner, or meal prep. Whether served as a standalone meal or as a side dish alongside grilled fish or roasted chicken, this quinoa pilaf is sure to become a favorite in your culinary repertoire.

Steamed Asparagus with Lemon Butter

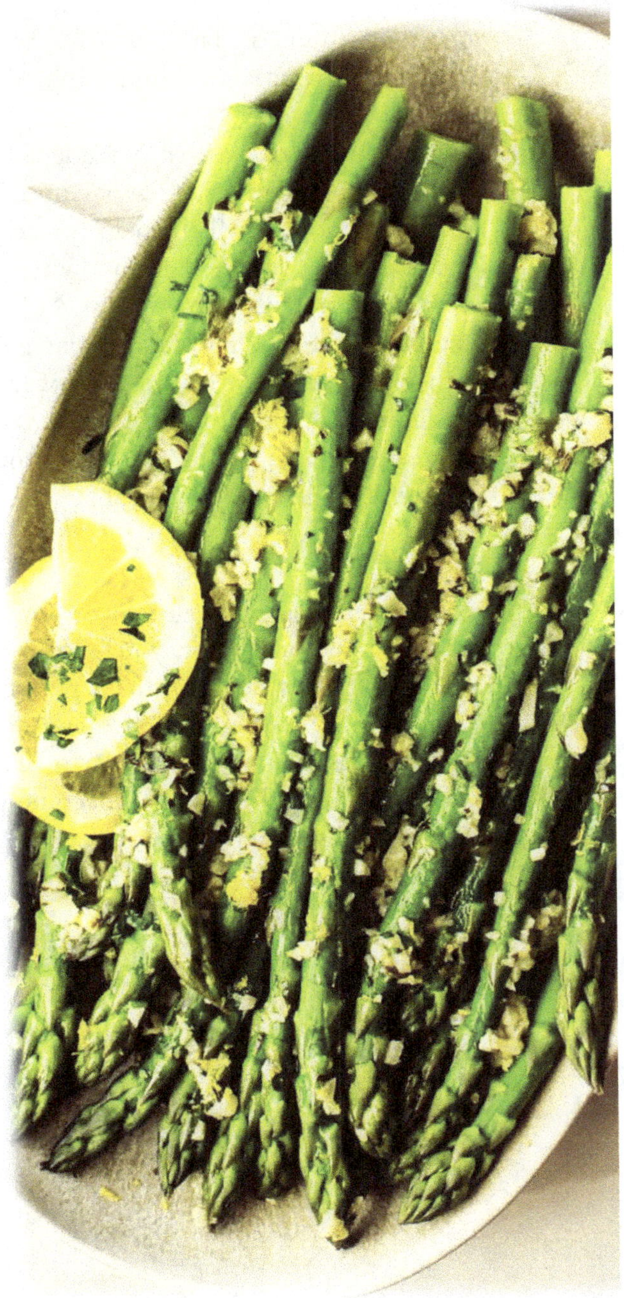

Ingredients:

- ❖ 1 bunch asparagus, trimmed
- ❖ 2 tablespoons unsalted butter
- ❖ 1 tablespoon freshly squeezed lemon juice
- ❖ Zest of 1 lemon
- ❖ Salt and pepper, to taste

Procedures:

- ❖ Fill a large pot with about an inch of water and bring it to a boil over high heat.
- ❖ Place a steamer basket or insert into the pot, making sure the water does not touch the bottom of the basket.
- ❖ Add the trimmed asparagus to the steamer basket, cover the pot, and steam for 3-5 minutes, or until the asparagus is tender but still crisp.
- ❖ While the asparagus is steaming, melt the unsalted butter in a small saucepan over low heat.
- ❖ Once melted, remove the saucepan from the heat and stir in the freshly squeezed lemon juice and lemon zest. Season with salt and pepper to taste.
- ❖ Once the asparagus is cooked, transfer it to a serving plate.
- ❖ Drizzle the lemon butter sauce over the steamed asparagus.
- ❖ Serve hot and enjoy!

- ❖ **Preparation Time:** 5 minutes
- ❖ **Cooking Time:** 5 minutes
- ❖ **Serving Unit:** 1 plate

Nutritional Values (per serving):

- ❖ **Calories:** 100
- ❖ **Protein:** 3g
- ❖ **Carbohydrates:** 7g
- ❖ **Dietary Fiber:** 4g
- ❖ **Sugars:** 2g

- ❖ **Fat**: 8g
- ❖ **Saturated Fat**: 5g
- ❖ **Cholesterol**: 20mg
- ❖ **Sodium**: 20mg
- ❖ **Potassium**: 350mg
- ❖ **Calcium**: 40mg
- ❖ **Iron**: 2mg

Cooking Tips:

- ❖ Choose fresh asparagus with firm, bright green spears and tight, compact tips for the best flavor and texture.
- ❖ Trim the tough ends of the asparagus by snapping them off where they naturally break or by cutting them with a knife.
- ❖ Avoid overcooking the asparagus, as it can become mushy and lose its vibrant color and flavor. Steam just until tender-crisp for the best results.
- ❖ Customize the lemon butter sauce by adding minced garlic, chopped fresh herbs (such as parsley or chives), or a pinch of red pepper flakes for extra flavor.
- ❖ For added richness, sprinkle freshly grated Parmesan cheese or toasted almond slices over the steamed asparagus before serving.

Health Benefits:

- ❖ **Nutrient-Rich:** Asparagus is a nutrient-rich vegetable, high in vitamins A, C, E, and K, as well as folate, potassium, and fiber, which support immune function, bone health, and overall well-being.
- ❖ **Low in Calories:** Asparagus is low in calories but high in fiber and water content, making it a satisfying and nutritious option for those watching their calorie intake.
- ❖ **Heart-Healthy Fats:** The unsalted butter used in the lemon butter sauce provides heart-healthy monounsaturated fats, which help reduce inflammation and improve cholesterol levels.
- ❖ **Rich in Antioxidants:** Asparagus is rich in antioxidants such as vitamin C and flavonoids, which help protect against oxidative stress and reduce the risk of chronic diseases.
- ❖ **Versatile and Flavorful:** Asparagus can be prepared in a variety of ways, including steaming, roasting, grilling, or sautéing, making it a versatile and flavorful addition to any meal.

By preparing this simple yet elegant Steamed Asparagus with Lemon Butter, you'll enjoy a delicious and nutritious side dish that's perfect for any occasion. Whether served alongside grilled salmon, roasted chicken, or as part of a vegetarian meal, this dish is sure to become a favorite in your culinary repertoire.

Baked Sweet Potato Fries

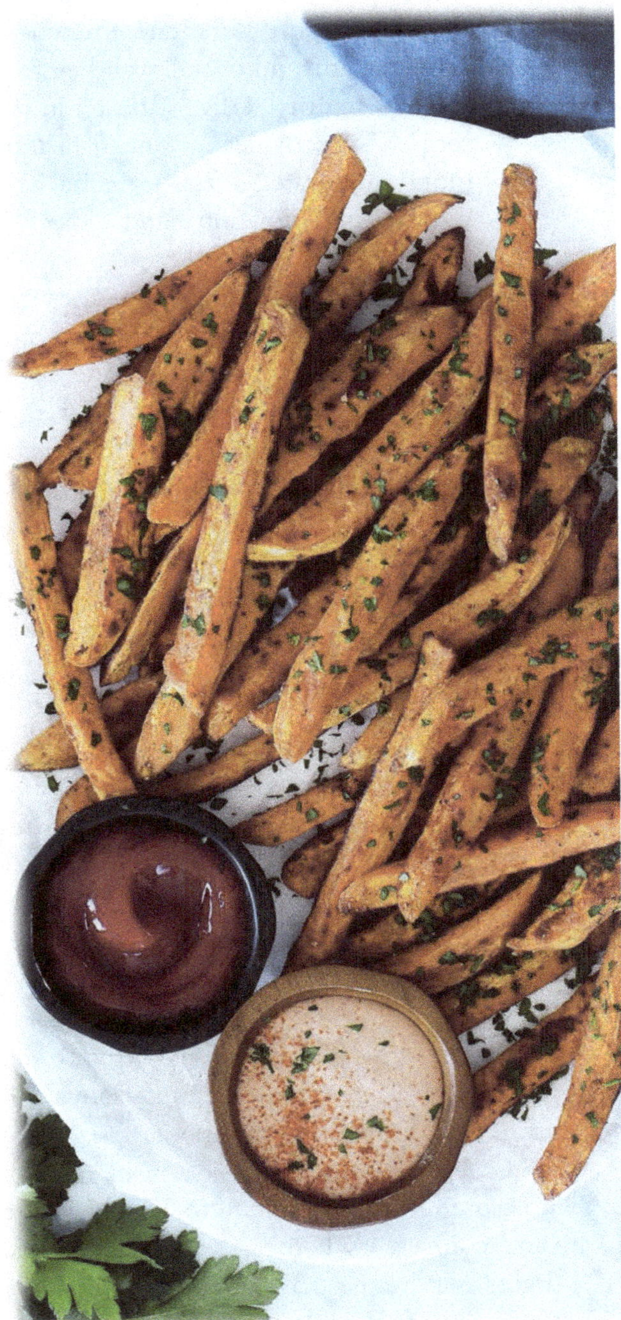

Ingredients:

- ❖ 2 medium sweet potatoes, sliced into fries after peeling.
- ❖ 2 tablespoons olive oil
- ❖ 1 teaspoon garlic powder
- ❖ 1 teaspoon paprika
- ❖ 1/2 teaspoon ground cumin
- ❖ 1/2 teaspoon chili powder (optional)
- ❖ Salt and pepper, to taste
- ❖ Garnish with optional fresh parsley or cilantro.

Procedures:

- ❖ Preheat the oven to 425°F (220°C) and line a baking sheet with parchment paper.
- ❖ In a large mixing bowl, toss the sweet potato fries with olive oil, garlic powder, paprika, ground cumin, and chili powder (if using) until evenly coated.
- ❖ Season the sweet potato fries with salt and pepper to taste, and toss again to combine.
- ❖ Spread the sweet potato fries in a single layer on the prepared baking sheet, making sure they are not touching or overlapping.
- ❖ Bake in the preheated oven for 20-25 minutes, or until the sweet potato fries are crispy and golden brown, flipping halfway through cooking.
- ❖ Once baked, remove the sweet potato fries from the oven and transfer them to a serving plate.
- ❖ Garnish with fresh parsley or cilantro, if desired.
- ❖ Serve hot and enjoy!

- ❖ **Preparation Time**: 10 minutes
- ❖ **Cooking Time**: 25 minutes
- ❖ **Serving Unit**: 1 plate

Nutritional Values (per serving):

- ❖ **Calories**: 200
- ❖ **Protein**: 2g
- ❖ **Carbohydrates**: 25g
- ❖ **Dietary Fiber**: 4g
- ❖ **Sugars**: 6g
- ❖ **Fat**: 10g
- ❖ **Saturated Fat**: 1g
- ❖ **Cholesterol**: 0mg
- ❖ **Sodium**: 200mg
- ❖ **Potassium**: 400mg
- ❖ **Calcium**: 40mg
- ❖ **Iron**: 1mg

Cooking Tips:

- ❖ Cut the sweet potato fries into uniform sizes to ensure even cooking.
- ❖ Soaking the cut sweet potato fries in cold water for 30 minutes before baking can help remove excess starch and make them crispier.
- ❖ Arrange the sweet potato fries in a single layer on the baking sheet with space between each fry to allow for proper airflow and even cooking.
- ❖ For extra crispiness, bake the sweet potato fries on a wire rack placed over the baking sheet.
- ❖ Avoid overcrowding the baking sheet, as this can cause the sweet potato fries to steam instead of crisp up.

Health Benefits:

- ❖ **Nutrient-Rich:** Sweet potatoes are rich in vitamins A, C, and E, as well as fiber, potassium, and antioxidants, which support immune function, vision health, and overall well-being.
- ❖ **Heart-Healthy: Olive** oil used in the recipe provides heart-healthy monounsaturated fats, which help reduce inflammation and improve cholesterol levels.
- ❖ **High in Fiber:** Sweet potatoes are high in dietary fiber, which promotes digestive health, regulates blood sugar levels, and supports weight management by promoting feelings of fullness and reducing hunger cravings.
- ❖ **Low in Calories:** Baked sweet potato fries are lower in calories and fat compared to traditional deep-fried fries, making them a healthier alternative for those watching their calorie intake.
- ❖ **Versatile and Flavorful:** Sweet potato fries can be seasoned with a variety of spices and herbs to suit different tastes and preferences, making them a versatile and flavorful side dish for any meal.

By preparing this simple yet flavorful Baked Sweet Potato Fries, you'll enjoy a delicious and nutritious alternative to traditional fries that's perfect for snacking, as a side dish, or as a wholesome accompaniment to your favorite main courses. Whether served alongside burgers, sandwiches, or grilled chicken, these sweet potato fries are sure to become a favorite in your meal rotation.

6

Introducing Hydrating Harmony: DASH Diet Beverage Bliss

Introducing Hydrating Harmony: DASH Diet Beverage Bliss

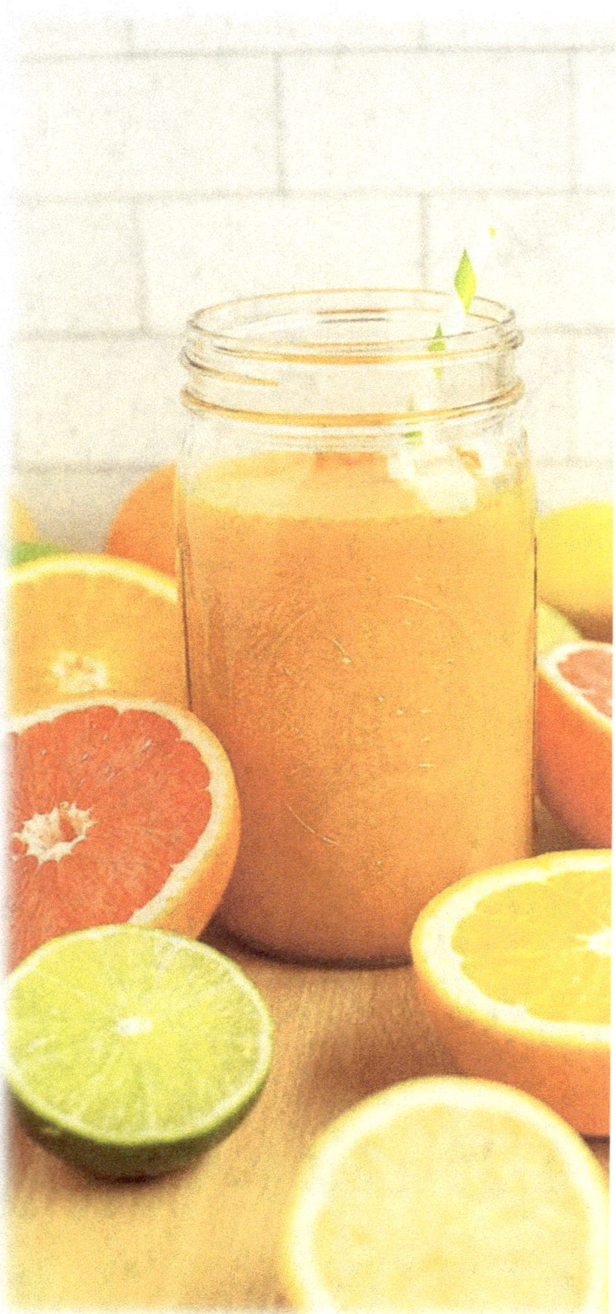

Welcome to "Hydrating Harmony: DASH Diet Beverage Bliss," where hydration meets health in a symphony of flavors and wellness. In this chapter, we explore the art of crafting beverages that not only quench your thirst but also align with the heart-healthy principles of the DASH (Dietary Approaches to Stop Hypertension) diet.

Join us as we journey through a refreshing world of drinks designed to invigorate your senses and elevate your hydration game. From vibrant smoothies bursting with fruits and vegetables to soothing herbal teas infused with aromatic spices, each recipe is thoughtfully crafted to provide hydration and nutritional benefits without compromising on taste.

Get ready to sip your way to wellness with "Hydrating Harmony: DASH Diet Beverage Bliss," where every sip brings you closer to your health goals and leaves you feeling refreshed, revitalized, and ready to take on the day. Cheers to hydration, health, and the joy of nourishing your body from the inside out!

Lemon Ginger Detox Water

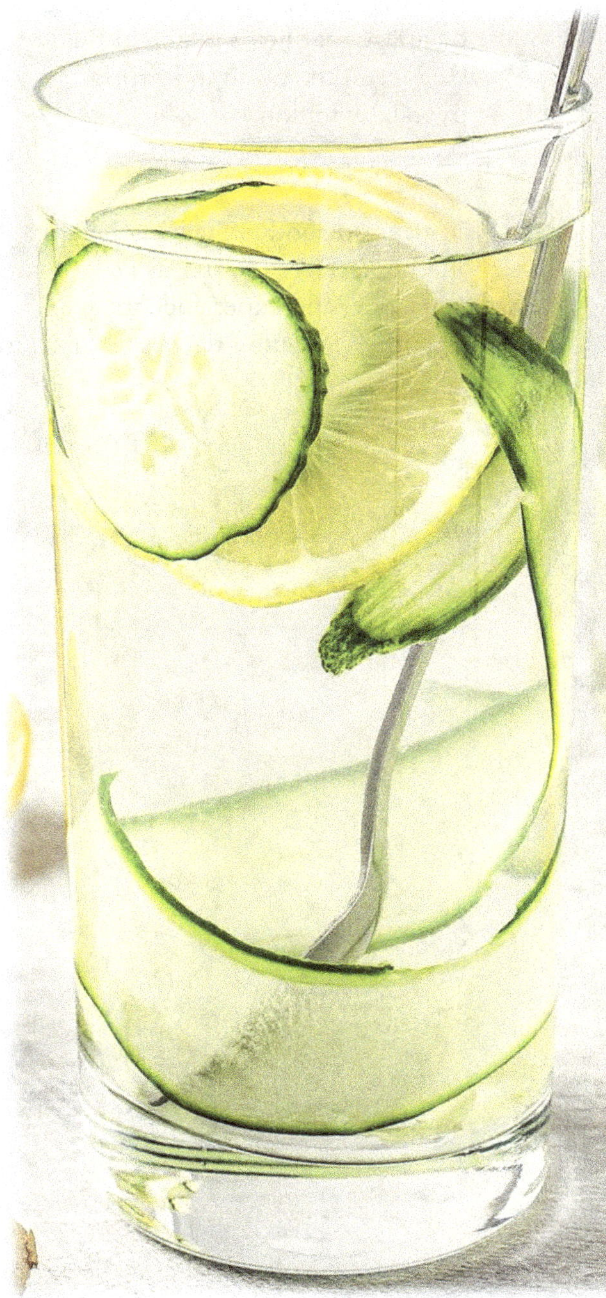

Ingredients:

* 1 lemon, thinly sliced
* 1-inch piece of fresh ginger, thinly sliced
* 6 cups water
* Fresh mint leaves (optional)
* Ice cubes (optional)

Procedures:

* Wash the lemon and ginger thoroughly under cold water.
* Slice the lemon and ginger into thin rounds or slices.
* Slices of ginger and lemon should be combined in a big pitcher.
* Pour 6 cups of water into the pitcher, covering the lemon and ginger completely.
* If desired, add a handful of fresh mint leaves to the pitcher for additional flavor.
* Add ice cubes to the pitcher to chill the water, if desired.
* Stir the ingredients gently to combine.
* Cover the pitcher and refrigerate for at least 1-2 hours to allow the flavors to infuse into the water.
* Once infused, pour the lemon ginger detox water into glasses, making sure to include some lemon and ginger slices in each glass.
* Serve chilled and enjoy the refreshing and cleansing properties of lemon ginger detox water!

* **Preparation Time:** 5 minutes
* **Serving Unit:** 1 pitcher

Nutritional Values (per serving):

* **Calories**: 0
* **Protein**: 0g
* **Carbohydrates**: 0g

- ❖ **Dietary Fiber**: 0g
- ❖ **Sugars**: 0g
- ❖ **Fat:** 0g
- ❖ **Saturated Fat:** 0g
- ❖ **Cholesterol:** 0mg
- ❖ **Sodium:** 0mg
- ❖ **Potassium:** 0mg

Cooking Tips:

- ❖ Use organic lemons and ginger whenever possible, especially if leaving the skin on, to minimize exposure to pesticides and chemicals.
- ❖ For a stronger flavor, gently crush the ginger slices before adding them to the pitcher to release their aromatic oils.
- ❖ Feel free to customize the detox water with additional ingredients such as cucumber slices, orange slices, or a pinch of cayenne pepper for added flavor and health benefits.
- ❖ Infuse the water for at least 1-2 hours to allow the flavors to develop fully. For a stronger infusion, let it sit in the refrigerator overnight.
- ❖ Keep the pitcher of detox water refrigerated and consume within 2-3 days for optimal freshness and flavor.

Health Benefits:

- ❖ **Detoxification:** Lemon and ginger are known for their detoxifying properties, helping to cleanse the body of toxins and promote liver health.
- ❖ **Digestive Aid:** Ginger aids digestion by stimulating the production of digestive enzymes and reducing nausea and bloating.
- ❖ **Immune Support:** The vitamin C in lemons and the anti-inflammatory properties of ginger help boost the immune system and protect against illness.
- ❖ **Hydration:** Lemon ginger detox water is a refreshing and hydrating beverage that helps maintain fluid balance in the body and supports overall hydration.

Enjoy the cleansing and revitalizing benefits of Lemon Ginger Detox Water as part of your hydration routine, and experience the refreshing and invigorating flavors it brings to your day.

Cucumber Mint Infused Water

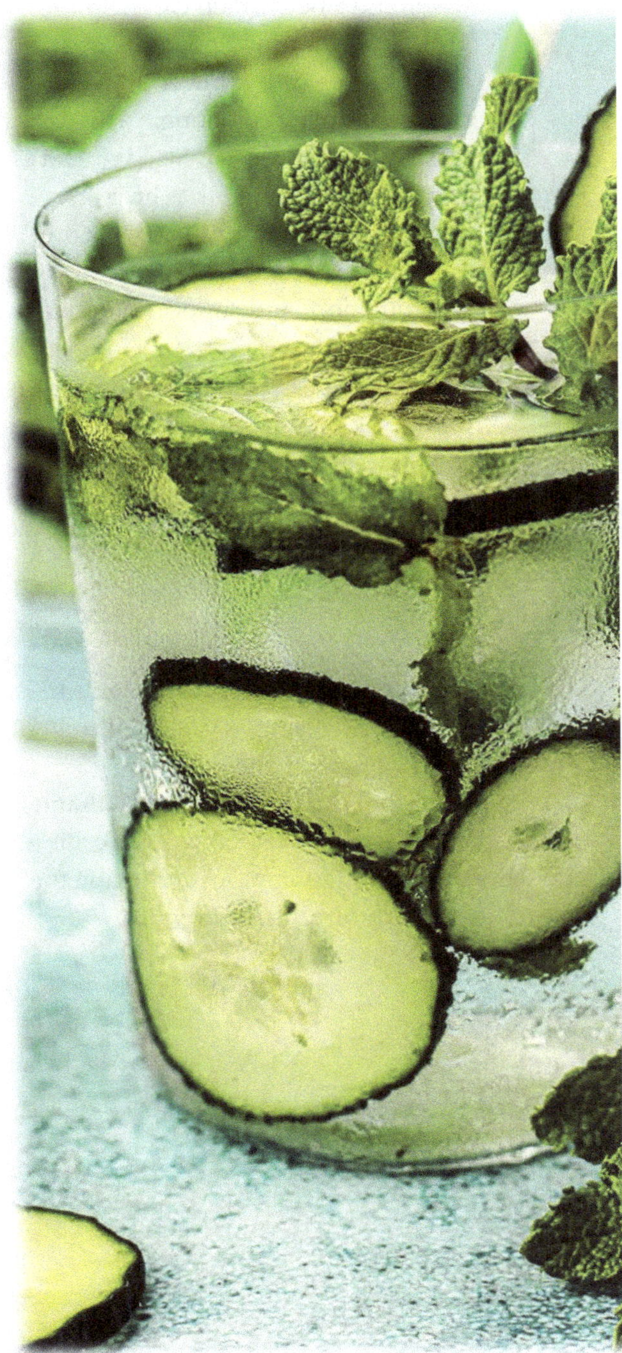

Ingredients:

- ❖ 1 cucumber, thinly sliced
- ❖ 10-12 fresh mint leaves
- ❖ 6 cups water
- ❖ Ice cubes (optional)

Procedures:

- ❖ After giving the cucumber a good wash, finely slice it. If desired, peel the cucumber before slicing.
- ❖ Rinse the fresh mint leaves under cold water and pat them dry with a paper towel.
- ❖ Add the mint leaves and cucumber slices to a big pitcher.
- ❖ Fill the pitcher with 6 cups of water, covering the cucumber slices and mint leaves completely.
- ❖ If you prefer a colder drink, add ice cubes to the pitcher.
- ❖ Stir the ingredients gently to combine.
- ❖ Cover the pitcher and refrigerate for at least 1-2 hours to allow the flavors to infuse into the water.
- ❖ After infusion, strain the cucumber-mint water into glasses, ensuring that each one has a few cucumber slices and mint leaves in it.
- ❖ Serve chilled and enjoy the refreshing taste of cucumber mint infused water!

- ❖ **Preparation Time:** 5 minutes
- ❖ **Serving Unit:** 1 pitcher

Nutritional Values (per serving):

- ❖ Calories: 0
- ❖ Protein: 0g
- ❖ Carbohydrates: 0g
- ❖ Dietary Fiber: 0g

❖ Sugars: 0g
❖ Fat: 0g
❖ Saturated Fat: 0g
❖ Cholesterol: 0mg
❖ Sodium: 0mg
❖ Potassium: 0mg

Cooking Tips:

❖ Use organic cucumbers whenever possible, especially if you plan to leave the skin on, to minimize exposure to pesticides and chemicals.
❖ For a stronger flavor, gently crush the mint leaves before adding them to the pitcher to release their aromatic oils.
❖ Feel free to customize the infused water with additional ingredients such as lemon slices, lime slices, or ginger for added flavor and health benefits.
❖ To enhance the flavor further, let the infused water sit in the refrigerator overnight for a more robust infusion of flavors.
❖ Refresh the pitcher of infused water with fresh cucumber slices and mint leaves every 1-2 days to maintain optimal flavor and freshness.
❖ Infused water can be kept refrigerated for up to 2-3 days. After this time, the flavor may begin to diminish, and the ingredients may start to break down.

Health Benefits:

❖ **Hydration:** Cucumber mint infused water is an excellent way to stay hydrated throughout the day, especially for those who find plain water boring or unappealing.
❖ **Refreshing:** The combination of cool cucumber and fresh mint creates a refreshing and invigorating drink that helps quench thirst and revitalize the senses.
❖ **Digestive Aid:** Cucumbers are rich in water and fiber, which can help promote hydration and support digestive health by preventing constipation and bloating.
❖ **Antioxidant Properties:** Mint leaves contain antioxidants that help neutralize free radicals in the body, reducing oxidative stress and inflammation, and supporting overall health.
❖ **Low-Calorie Alternative:** Infused water is naturally calorie-free and contains no added sugars or artificial sweeteners, making it a healthy and refreshing alternative to sugary beverages.

the crisp and revitalizing flavor of cucumber mint infused water, a simple yet delightful beverage that nourishes the body and refreshes the soul. Incorporate this hydrating drink into your daily routine for a refreshing boost of flavor and hydration, and enjoy the numerous health benefits it provides.

Turmeric Ginger Tea

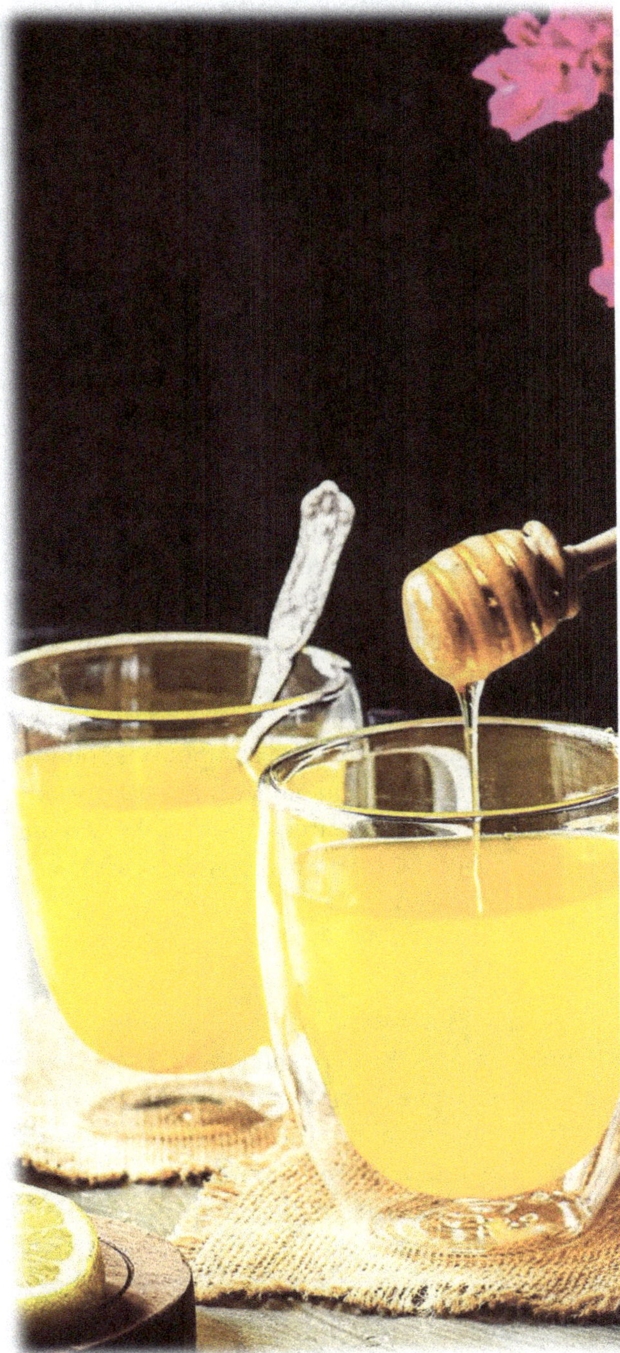

Ingredients:

- ❖ A tablespoon of freshly grated turmeric or one teaspoon of crushed turmeric
- ❖ 1 teaspoon grated fresh ginger
- ❖ 2 cups water
- ❖ 1 teaspoon honey or maple syrup (optional)
- ❖ Juice of half a lemon (optional)

Procedures:

- ❖ In a small saucepan, combine the ground or grated turmeric, grated ginger, and water.
- ❖ Bring the mixture to a boil over medium heat, then reduce the heat to low and simmer for 5-10 minutes, allowing the flavors to infuse into the water.
- ❖ Remove the saucepan from the heat and let the tea cool slightly.
- ❖ Strain the tea through a fine-mesh sieve or tea strainer into a cup.
- ❖ If desired, stir in honey or maple syrup to sweeten the tea, and add a squeeze of lemon juice for extra flavor.
- ❖ Serve the turmeric ginger tea hot and enjoy its soothing and invigorating properties!

Nutritional Values (per serving):

- ❖ **Calories**: 15
- ❖ **Protein**: 0g
- ❖ **Carbohydrates**: 4g
- ❖ **Dietary Fiber**: 1g
- ❖ **Sugars**: 2g
- ❖ **Fat**: 0g
- ❖ **Saturated Fat**: 0g
- ❖ **Cholesterol**: 0mg

- ❖ **Preparation Time:** 5 minutes
- ❖ **Cooking Time:** 10 minutes
- ❖ **Serving Unit:** 1 cup

❖ **Sodium:** 10mg
❖ **Potassium:** 200mg
❖ **Vitamin C:** 10mg
❖ **Iron:** 0.5mg

Cooking Tips:

❖ Use fresh turmeric and ginger whenever possible for the best flavor and health benefits. Simply peel the turmeric and ginger roots and grate them using a fine grater or microplane.

❖ Adjust the amount of turmeric and ginger according to your taste preferences. If you prefer a stronger flavor, add more turmeric and ginger to the tea.

❖ Fresh turmeric stains clothes and surfaces, so handle it with caution. Use gloves or wash your hands immediately after handling to prevent staining.

❖ If you don't have fresh ginger on hand, you can substitute with ground ginger, although fresh ginger offers a more vibrant flavor and aroma.

❖ Feel free to customize the tea with additional ingredients such as cinnamon, black pepper, or cloves for added warmth and spice.

❖ Store any leftover turmeric ginger tea in the refrigerator for up to 2-3 days. Reheat gently on the stove or in the microwave before serving.

Health Benefits:

❖ **Anti-Inflammatory Properties:** Both turmeric and ginger contain potent anti-inflammatory compounds, such as curcumin and gingerol, which help reduce inflammation in the body and alleviate symptoms of inflammatory conditions like arthritis and joint pain.

❖ **Digestive Aid:** Ginger is well-known for its digestive benefits, helping to alleviate nausea, indigestion, and bloating. Turmeric also supports digestive health by stimulating bile production and improving gut function.

❖ **Immune Support:** Turmeric and ginger are rich in antioxidants and antimicrobial compounds that help strengthen the immune system and protect against infections and illnesses.

❖ **Heart Health:** Turmeric and ginger have been linked to improved heart health by reducing cholesterol levels, lowering blood pressure, and preventing blood clot formation, thus reducing the risk of heart disease.

❖ **Mood Enhancement:** Some research suggests that the compounds found in turmeric and ginger may have mood-enhancing effects, potentially helping alleviate symptoms of depression and anxiety.

Indulge in the soothing and invigorating properties of turmeric ginger tea, a warm and comforting beverage that nourishes the body and calms the mind. Incorporate this flavorful tea into your daily routine to enjoy its numerous health benefits and promote overall well-being.

Citrus Sunshine Juice

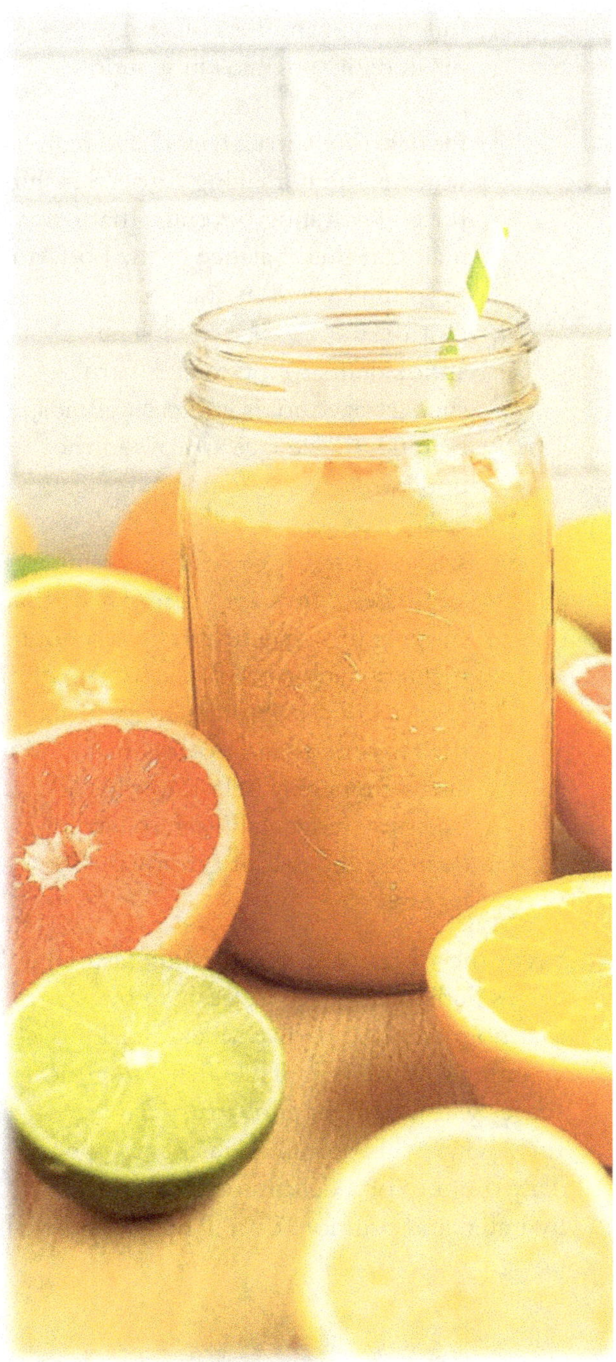

Ingredients:

- ❖ 1 orange, peeled and segmented
- ❖ 1 grapefruit, peeled and segmented
- ❖ Juice of 1/2 lemon
- ❖ 1 teaspoon honey or maple syrup (optional)
- ❖ Ice cubes (optional)

Procedures:

- ❖ Prepare the citrus fruits by peeling and segmenting the orange and grapefruit. Ensure that no seeds or pith remain.
- ❖ Place the orange segments, grapefruit segments, and lemon juice into a blender or juicer.
- ❖ If desired, add honey or maple syrup to sweeten the juice. You may change the sweetness to suit your own tastes.
- ❖ Blend or juice the citrus fruits until smooth and well-combined.
- ❖ If you prefer a colder drink, add ice cubes to the blender or pour the juice over ice in a glass.
- ❖ Once blended, pour the Citrus Sunshine Juice into a glass.
- ❖ Garnish with a slice of orange or grapefruit, if desired.
- ❖ Serve immediately and enjoy the refreshing and invigorating taste of Citrus Sunshine Juice!

Nutritional Values (per serving):

- ❖ **Calories:** 80
- ❖ **Protein:** 2g
- ❖ **Carbohydrates:** 20g
- ❖ **Dietary Fiber:** 4g
- ❖ **Sugars:** 14g
- ❖ **Fat:** 0g

- ❖ **Preparation Time:** 10 minutes
- ❖ Serving Unit: 1 glass

- ❖ **Saturated Fat**: 0g
- ❖ **Cholesterol**: 0mg
- ❖ **Sodium**: 0mg
- ❖ **Potassium**: 300mg
- ❖ **Vitamin C**: 120mg

Cooking Tips:

- ❖ Use ripe and juicy citrus fruits for the best flavor and juiciness. Look for fruits that are heavy for their size and have smooth, firm skin.
- ❖ Feel free to mix and match different citrus fruits according to your preferences. You can use blood oranges, tangerines, or pomelos in addition to or instead of oranges and grapefruits.
- ❖ To extract the maximum juice from the citrus fruits, roll them on the countertop with gentle pressure before cutting and juicing.
- ❖ For a smoother juice, strain the blended mixture through a fine-mesh sieve or cheesecloth to remove any pulp or fibers.
- ❖ Customize the juice with additional ingredients such as ginger, mint, or a splash of sparkling water for added flavor and fizz.
- ❖ Enjoy the Citrus Sunshine Juice immediately after preparing to experience its vibrant and refreshing taste at its best.

- ❖ **Rich in Vitamin C:** Citrus fruits are a powerhouse of vitamin C, an essential nutrient that supports immune function, promotes collagen production, and aids in wound healing.
- ❖ **Hydration:** Citrus fruits have high water content, making Citrus Sunshine Juice a hydrating beverage that helps maintain fluid balance in the body and supports overall hydration.
- ❖ **Antioxidant Properties:** The antioxidants found in citrus fruits, such as flavonoids and carotenoids, help neutralize free radicals in the body, reducing oxidative stress and inflammation.
- ❖ **Digestive Aid:** Citrus fruits contain natural enzymes and dietary fiber that support digestive health by promoting regularity and preventing constipation.
- ❖ **Heart Health:** Studies suggest that the flavonoids and potassium found in citrus fruits may help lower blood pressure, reduce cholesterol levels, and decrease the risk of cardiovascular disease.

Savor the vibrant and invigorating taste of Citrus Sunshine Juice, a refreshing beverage that nourishes the body with essential vitamins and minerals while delighting the senses with its bright and citrusy flavor. Incorporate this nutritious juice into your daily routine for a delicious way to stay hydrated and promote overall health and well-being.

Health Benefits:

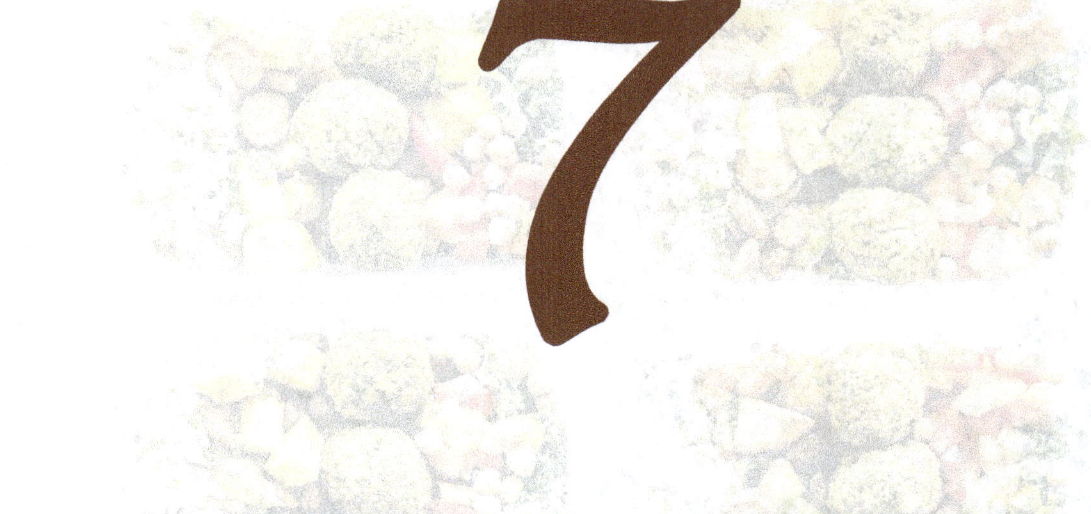

7

Introduction to Meal Planning

Introduction to Meal Planning

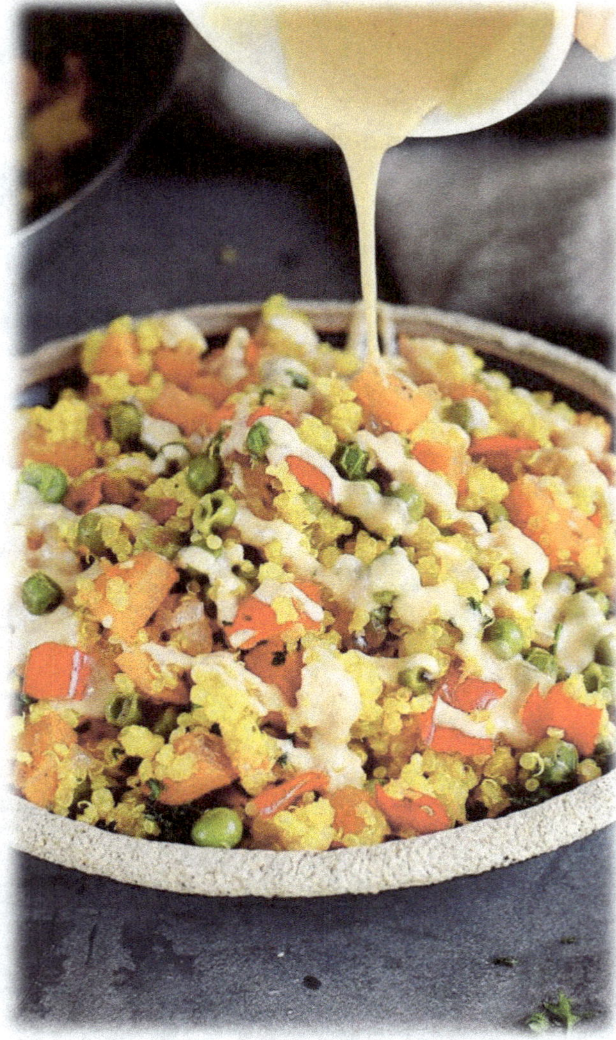

Meal planning is a proactive approach to organizing and preparing meals ahead of time, typically for a specified period, such as a week or a month. It involves deciding what to eat, creating a shopping list, and preparing ingredients or even full meals in advance. A well-thought-out meal plan can help individuals and families save time, money, and stress while promoting healthier eating habits and reducing food waste.

Meal planning offers numerous benefits, including:

- ❖ **Healthier Eating:** By planning meals in advance, you can ensure that your diet is balanced and nutritious, incorporating a variety of fruits, vegetables, whole grains, lean proteins, and healthy fats.
- ❖ **Time-Saving:** Meal planning streamlines the cooking process by eliminating the need to decide what to make each day. With meals planned out, you can spend less time in the kitchen during busy weekdays.
- ❖ **Cost-Effective:** Planning meals allows you to make more efficient use of ingredients, reducing the likelihood of impulse purchases and minimizing food waste. Over time, this may result in considerable cost savings.
- ❖ **Reduced Stress:** Knowing what you'll be eating for the week ahead can alleviate the stress of last-minute meal decisions. It can also help avoid the temptation of unhealthy convenience foods on hectic days.
- ❖ **Customization:** Meal planning allows you to tailor your meals to meet specific dietary preferences, restrictions, or health goals, whether you're following a specific diet plan or accommodating food allergies.

Meal planning is a practical tool for promoting a healthier lifestyle, saving time and money, and reducing the stress associated with mealtime decisions. With careful planning and organization, anyone can enjoy the benefits of a well-executed meal plan.

Day 1:
Breakfast: Quinoa Breakfast Bowl
Lunch: Mediterranean Chickpea Salad
Dinner: Baked Sweet Potato Fries

Day 2:
Breakfast: Berry Blast Smoothie
Lunch: Turkey and Avocado Wrap
Dinner: Quinoa Pilaf with Mixed Vegetables

Day 3:
Breakfast: Veggie-Packed Omelette
Lunch: Zucchini Noodles with Pesto
Dinner: Steamed Asparagus with Lemon Butter

Day 4:
Breakfast: Whole Wheat Pancakes with Fresh Fruit
Lunch: Hummus and Veggie Sticks
Dinner: Caprese Salad with Balsamic Glaze

Day 5:
Breakfast: Quinoa Breakfast Bowl
Lunch: Mediterranean Chickpea Salad
Dinner: Butternut Squash Soup

Day 6:
Breakfast: Berry Blast Smoothie
Lunch: Turkey and Avocado Wrap
Dinner: Greek Yogurt with Berries

Day 7:
Breakfast: Veggie-Packed Omelette
Lunch: Zucchini Noodles with Pesto
Dinner: Minestrone Soup

Day 8:
Breakfast: Whole Wheat Pancakes with Fresh Fruit

Lunch: Hummus and Veggie Sticks
Dinner: Cucumber and Tomato Slices with Feta

Day 9:
Breakfast: Quinoa Breakfast Bowl
Lunch: Mediterranean Chickpea Salad
Dinner: Kale Caesar Salad with Grilled Chicken

Day 10:
Breakfast: Berry Blast Smoothie
Lunch: Turkey and Avocado Wrap
Dinner: Homemade Trail Mix

Day 11:
Breakfast: Veggie-Packed Omelette
Lunch: Zucchini Noodles with Pesto
Dinner: Minestrone Soup

Day 12:
Breakfast: Whole Wheat Pancakes with Fresh Fruit
Lunch: Hummus and Veggie Sticks
Dinner: Caprese Salad with Balsamic Glaze

Day 13:
Breakfast: Quinoa Breakfast Bowl
Lunch: Mediterranean Chickpea Salad
Dinner: Butternut Squash Soup

Day 14:
Breakfast: Berry Blast Smoothie
Lunch: Turkey and Avocado Wrap
Dinner: Greek Yogurt with Berries

Day 15:
Breakfast: Veggie-Packed Omelette
Lunch: Zucchini Noodles with Pesto
Dinner: Cucumber and Tomato Slices with Feta

Day 16:
Breakfast: Quinoa Breakfast Bowl
Lunch: Mediterranean Chickpmmea Salad

Dinner: Kale Caesar Salad with Grilled Chicken
Day 17:
Breakfast: Berry Blast Smoothie
Lunch: Turkey and Avocado Wrap
Dinner: Homemade Trail Mix
Day 18:
Breakfast: Veggie-Packed Omelette
Lunch: Zucchini Noodles with Pesto
Dinner: Steamed Asparagus with Lemon Butter
Day 19:
Breakfast: Whole Wheat Pancakes with Fresh Fruit
Lunch: Hummus and Veggie Sticks
Dinner: Caprese Salad with Balsamic Glaze
Day 20:
Breakfast: Quinoa Breakfast Bowl
Lunch: Mediterranean Chickpea Salad
Dinner: Butternut Squash Soup!
Day 21:
Breakfast: Berry Blast Smoothie
Lunch: Turkey and Avocado Wrap
Dinner: Greek Yogurt with Berries
Day 22:
Breakfast: Veggie-Packed Omelette
Lunch: Zucchini Noodles with Pesto
Dinner: Minestrone Soup
Day 23:
Breakfast: Whole Wheat Pancakes with Fresh Fruit
Lunch: Hummus and Veggie Sticks
Dinner: Cucumber and Tomato Slices with Feta
Day 24:
Breakfast: Quinoa Breakfast Bowl
Lunch: Mediterranean Chickpea Salad

Dinner: Kale Caesar Salad with Grilled Chicken
Day 25:
Breakfast: Berry Blast Smoothie
Lunch: Turkey and Avocado Wrap
Dinner: Homemade Trail Mix
Day 26:
Breakfast: Veggie-Packed Omelette
Lunch: Zucchini Noodles with Pesto
Dinner: Steamed Asparagus with Lemon Butter
Day 27:
Breakfast: Whole Wheat Pancakes with Fresh Fruit
Lunch: Hummus and Veggie Sticks
Dinner: Caprese Salad with Balsamic Glaze
Day 28:
Breakfast: Quinoa Breakfast Bowl
Lunch: Mediterranean Chickpea Salad
Dinner: Butternut Squash Soup
Day 29:
Breakfast: Berry Blast Smoothie
Lunch: Turkey and Avocado Wrap
Dinner: Greek Yogurt with Berries
Day 30:
Breakfast: Veggie-Packed Omelette
Lunch: Zucchini Noodles with Pesto
Dinner: Minestrone Soup

This 30-day meal plan provides a variety of nutritious and delicious meals using the recipes provided. Feel free to adjust the plan to suit your preferences and dietary needs. Enjoy your meals!

Conclusion

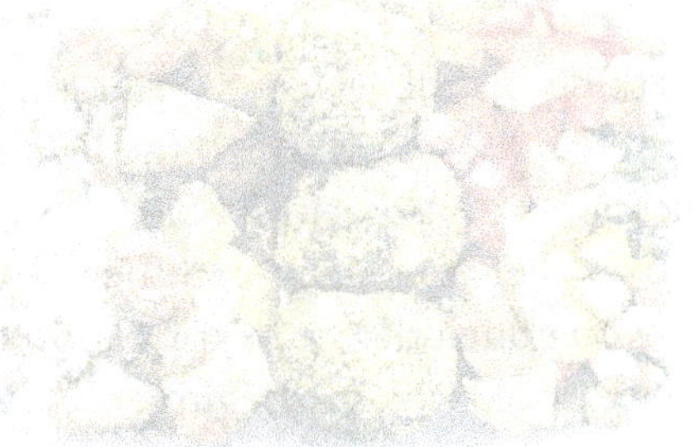

Conclusion

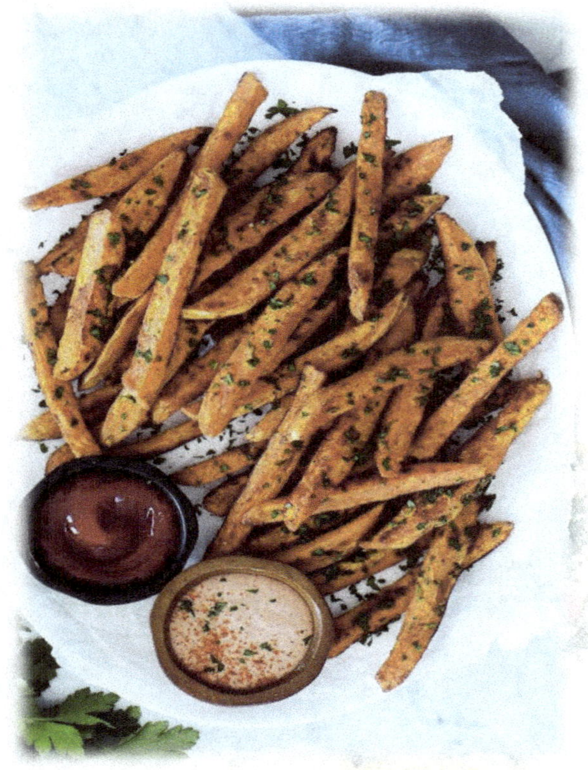

As you've journeyed through the pages of this cookbook, you've discovered a plethora of recipes designed to tantalize your palate while aligning with the heart-healthy guidelines of the DASH diet. From vibrant breakfast bowls and wholesome salads to comforting soups and flavorful main courses, each recipe has offered a culinary adventure, inviting you to savor the goodness of fresh, whole foods.

Moreover, you've honed your culinary skills, mastering techniques to prepare delicious and nutritious meals with ease. Whether you're sautéing vegetables, roasting meats, or blending smoothies, you've embraced the joy of cooking, transforming simple ingredients into culinary delights that nourish both body and soul.

Embarking on the journey of adopting a healthier lifestyle through the DASH (Dietary Approaches to Stop Hypertension) diet is a commendable endeavor. As you conclude your exploration of the DASH Diet Cookbook for Beginners 2024, it's essential to reflect on the valuable knowledge and culinary skills you've acquired.

As you bid farewell to this cookbook, remember that your journey towards better health and well-being is ongoing. While the recipes provided serve as a foundation for your culinary endeavors, feel empowered to experiment, innovate, and tailor your meals to suit your taste preferences and dietary needs. Embrace the principles of the DASH diet as a guide for making mindful food choices, prioritizing whole, nutrient-rich foods while minimizing processed and unhealthy options. Cultivate a love for cooking and nourishing your body, recognizing that every meal is an opportunity to fuel yourself with the goodness of nature's bounty.

Through this cookbook, you've delved into the intricacies of the DASH diet, gaining a deeper understanding of its principles and benefits. You've learned how to incorporate nutrient-rich ingredients into your meals, crafting dishes that not only tantalize your taste buds but also nourish your body and support your overall well-being.

Bon appétit, and here's to your continued success on your journey towards optimal health and vitality!

www.ingramcontent.com/pod-product-compliance
Lightning Source LLC
Chambersburg PA
CBHW081600250726
48653CB00009B/3521